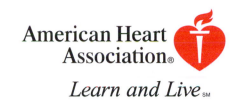

American Heart
Association®

Learn and Live SM

HEARTSAVER®
FIRST AID WITH
CPR and AED

STUDENT WORKBOOK

ISBN 0-87493-478-8
© 2006 American Heart Association

Contents

CD Contents

Preface

As a cofounder of the National First Aid Science Advisory Board, the American Heart Association (AHA) is dedicated to helping to reduce the number of deaths due to emergency events. With the basic first aid you will learn in this course, you could make a difference in the lives of others. You might even save the life of someone you know.

The single most important thing you need to know as a first aid rescuer is how and when to get help if needed. The AHA adult Chain of Survival focuses on calling your emergency response number (or 911) and early access to medical care.

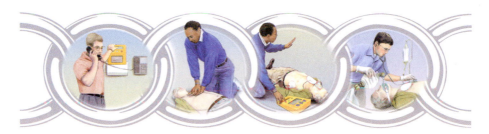

The members of the AHA First Aid Task Force have been instrumental in developing this course. Their outstanding efforts underscore the AHA's commitment to providing exceptional first aid education to people around the world.

William W. Hammill, MD
First Aid Task Force Chair

Considerations for International Readers

The following table is intended for international participants of this course. It is meant to help explain materials in this course that may be relevant only to those in the United States. For more specific information about your local practices and organizations, please contact your instructor.

Page 7	The Occupational Safety and Health Administration (OSHA) is a US organization. Please contact your local authority for the safety and health standards for your workplace.
Page 71	The coral snake is native to the US. Please talk to your instructor about poisonous snakes in your area.
Page 73	The black widow spider and the brown recluse spider are given as examples of poisonous spiders. These spiders are native to the US. Please talk to your instructor about poisonous insects and spiders in your area.
Page 84	In the section **Actions for Poison Emergencies,** the telephone number for the US National Poison Control Center (800-222-1222) is for the US only. Please ask your instructor for the poison control number in your area.
Page 91	In step 5 of the section **Actions for Chest Compressions,** please note the following metric conversion: 1½ to 2 inches = 4 to 5 cm
Page 107	In the box **FYI: AEDs in the Community,** please consult with your instructor regarding the placement of AEDs and organizations supporting the public placement of AEDs in your region.

Introduction

Overview

This student workbook gives you first aid basics. As you use this student workbook, remember that you don't have to make all the decisions. We will tell you how and when to get help if you need it.

Who Should Take This Course

We wrote this course for anyone who needs to learn basic first aid.

How This Course Is Organized

You will learn first aid basics through this student workbook and the video for the course. After each section of the course, you will answer a few written test questions.

During the course you will practice some skills. If you demonstrate that you can do the skills taught in the course, you will receive a Heartsaver First Aid card.

Using This Student Workbook

This student workbook is both a classroom textbook and a workbook. You should use this student workbook in the following ways:

When	Then you should
Before the course	• Read this student workbook and look at the pictures on each page. • Watch the video clips on the CD. This will help you learn the important points and prepare for practice during the course.
During the course	• Use this student workbook to understand the important information and skills taught in the course. • Take notes about your group's policies and procedures. For example, if you work in a facility that has established policies and procedures for emergencies, review these documents and take notes about how this information will apply to you.
After the course	• Review the skills frequently. Look at the practice sheets in the student workbook or the video skills on the CD. This will help you remember the steps of first aid, CPR, and automated external defibrillator (AED) use. You'll always be ready if there is an emergency.

Using the Student CD

More information is available on the CD (included with this student workbook). You should use the student CD in the following ways:

When	Then you should
Before the course	• Watch the video clips. This will help you learn the important points and prepare for practice during the course.
After the course	• View the video clips after class as a review. • Review the reference materials and other information on the CD.

See the list of CD contents on page iv.

Heartsaver First Aid Quick Reference Guide

The Heartsaver First Aid Quick Reference Guide summarizes first aid actions for many injuries and illnesses. Use this to help you remember how to give first aid after you take this course.

How Often Training Is Needed

Review your student workbook, student CD, and quick reference guide often to keep your skills fresh. You need to retake this course every 2 years to get a new course completion card.

Icons

These icons will help you as you use this student workbook.

Icon	Meaning
	Go online for more information about this topic.
	Check the student CD for more information about this topic.

First Aid Basics

Case Example

Your company has asked you to learn how to give first aid. As you get ready to take the course, some questions cross your mind:

- What is first aid?
- Do I have to help? What is my responsibility?
- Will I get into legal trouble if I make a mistake?
- Will I remember what I have learned? Will I be able to act in an emergency?

What You Will Learn

By the end of this section you should be able to

- Tell what first aid is
- Tell who has a duty to give first aid
- Tell where to find a list of items in the first aid kit at your worksite

What First Aid Is

First aid is the *immediate* care that you give someone with an illness or injury *before* trained help arrives and takes over. Trained help could be someone whose job is taking care of people who are ill or injured such as an EMS responder, nurse, or doctor.

Your actions during the first minutes of an emergency can be critical. What *you* do may help a victim recover more completely or more quickly.

Most of the time you will give first aid for minor illnesses or injuries. But you may also be called upon to give first aid for a serious illness or injury, such as a heart attack or major bleeding.

The first aid that you provide may mean the difference between life and death. Or it may mean the difference between a quick recovery and a long illness. *You* can make a difference!

Responsibility to Provide First Aid

If you drive past a car crash, *you* can decide whether to stop and help. If you are walking down the street and see a person who seems ill, *you* can decide if you will help. The choice is yours.

But if giving first aid is part of your job description, you *must* help while you are working. You may be assigned to give first aid in addition to your other work, or it may be part of your job description. Law enforcement officers, firefighters, flight attendants, lifeguards, and park rangers have a duty to give first aid when they are working. But even they can decide whether to stop and help when they are off duty.

Duty to Act

You have a duty to give the level of care that you will learn in this first aid course. You have a legal responsibility to act the way a reasonable person with your level of training would act. No one expects you to give the level of care given by a professional such as an EMS rescuer, a nurse, a physician, or other healthcare worker.

If it is your duty to respond, you should offer to help. The victim may accept or refuse your offer.

Follow these steps when you find an ill or injured person who may need first aid:

Step	Action
1	If the victim responds, introduce yourself before you touch him/her: *"My name is Joe Smith and I am trained in first aid. May I help you?"*
2	If the victim agrees, you may give first aid.
3	If the victim refuses your help, phone your company's emergency response number (or 911), and stay with the victim until trained help arrives and takes over.
4	If the victim is confused or cannot answer, assume that he or she would want you to help.

Will I Remember What I Have Learned? Will I Be Able to Act in an Emergency?

This course will teach you how to recognize an emergency and what to do. But if you don't use or practice your skills often, you will forget them. We all forget things that we don't use often.

To be prepared to help in a real emergency, you must learn the material and practice the skills. Then every 1 or 2 months you should review and practice what you have learned. Use this workbook to help you review.

> **Important**
>
> Remember: Review and practice your skills often. If you don't use or practice your skills, you may forget them.

The First Aid Kit

The first aid kit contains supplies that you might need in an emergency.

- ■ Keep the supplies in a sturdy, water-tight container that is clearly labeled.
- ■ Know where the first aid kit is.
- ■ Replace what you use so the kit will be ready for the next emergency.
- ■ Check the kit often to make sure it is complete and ready for an emergency.

Not all first aid kits contain the same supplies. Your company will decide what supplies the first aid kit should contain. The Appendix to this section (on page 18) lists sample supplies that might be useful in a first aid kit.

Victim and Rescuer Safety

"Dead heroes can't save lives. Injured heroes are a nuisance. So check the scene for hazards before you lurch in."

— Nancy L. Caroline, *Emergency Care in the Streets*

Case Example

A truck has struck an employee in the parking lot. You see a man lying on the ground. Several co-workers have gathered around him. You note that traffic is moving slowly around the crash.

Would you know what to do?

What You Will Learn

By the end of this section you should be able to

- ■ Tell how to keep yourself safe when giving first aid
- ■ Tell how to keep the victim from further injury when giving first aid
- ■ Show how to put on and take off protective gloves

Scene Safety

You may have to give first aid in dangerous places. The victim may be in a room with poisonous fumes, on a busy street, or in a company parking lot. You and others near the victim(s) will be nervous and excited, especially if you know the victim. You will have to make important decisions. You may not be thinking about harm or injury to yourself.

Remember: *You must not put yourself in danger while trying to help others. You could become a victim when you are trying to be a rescuer. Always look around and check for safety—safety for yourself and safety for the victim!*

Always look around and make sure the scene is safe for you and the victim **first** (Figure 1). Do not waste time. Look around as you approach the victim.

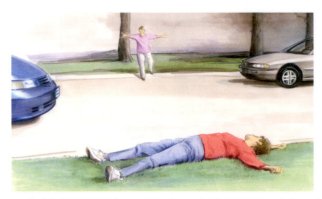

Figure 1. Make sure the scene is safe for you and the victim.

What Are You Looking For?

As you approach the scene, you should think about the following:

- **■** *Is there any danger for the rescuer?* Sometimes rescuers are injured while trying to provide first aid. Watch your footing. Watch where you are going. Do not attempt a dangerous act. Examples of acts that might be dangerous include crossing many lanes of a busy interstate highway or entering an area with spilled gasoline or downed power lines.

- **■** *Is there any danger for the victim?* As a rule, do not move an ill or injured victim. Move a victim only if the scene is unsafe or if it is necessary to provide first aid or CPR (eg, the victim is facedown and does not respond, or the victim is vomiting). If you do have to move a victim from danger, such as a fire or collapsing building, use one of the methods shown (Figure 2).

- **■** *Are there other people around who can help?* Ask others to direct traffic and phone your company's emergency response number (or 911). That way you can begin to give first aid to the victim.

- **■** *Where is the nearest telephone? Does anyone have a cellular phone?* Ask someone to phone your company's emergency response number (or 911).

- **■** *How many people are injured? How were they injured?* Look around to be sure you see everyone who might need help. Try to get an idea of what happened.

- **■** *What is your location?* Address, floor, location in building or on the property.

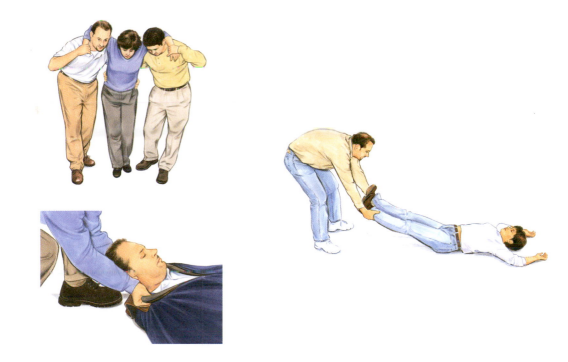

Figure 2. If a victim is in danger, use one of these methods to move the victim.

FYI: Know Your Limits

When you give first aid, know your limits. Don't become another victim. Sometimes your wish to help can put you in danger. For example, if you are not a good swimmer, you must be very careful when you try to save a drowning victim.

Protection From Blood-Borne Diseases

This section is based on recommendations of the Occupational Safety and Health Administration (OSHA).

Body fluids, such as blood, saliva, and urine, can sometimes carry germs that cause diseases. Whenever you give first aid you should

■ Use personal protective equipment provided by your employer. Throughout this workbook we will assume that you use personal protective equipment whenever the equipment is available. Personal protective equipment (Figure 3) includes

— Gloves to protect your hands from blood and other body fluids
— Eye protection, if the victim is bleeding, to protect your eyes from blood and other body fluids
— Mask to protect you when you give breaths (see section on CPR)

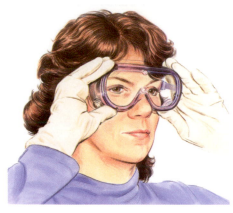

Figure 3. Wear protective gloves whenever you give first aid and wear eye protection if a victim is bleeding.

■ Place all disposable equipment that has touched body fluids in a biohazard waste bag (if required by your workplace) and seal it (Figure 4). *Don't throw the biohazard waste bag in the trash.* Follow your company's plan for disposing of hazardous waste.

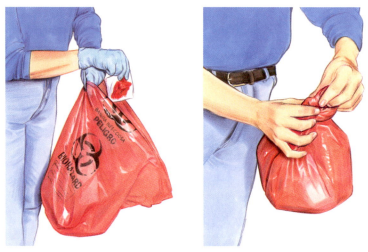

Figure 4. Place all disposable equipment that has touched body fluids in a biohazard waste bag if one is available, and seal it.

■ Wash your hands *well* with soap and water after properly taking off your gloves (Figure 5).

Figure 5. Wash your hands well with soap and water after properly taking off your gloves.

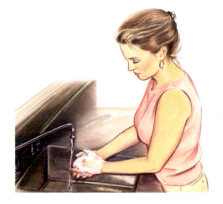

These steps are called "universal precautions": *"Universal"* because you should treat *everyone* as if he or she were infected and *"precautions"* because they are intended to *protect* you and your co-workers.

FYI: Latex Allergies

Some rescuers and victims may be allergic to latex. Use protective gloves that don't contain latex, for example, vinyl gloves, whenever possible.

If you or the victim has a latex allergy, do not use gloves that contain latex.

If you have a latex allergy, tell your emergency response program supervisor and your Heartsaver First Aid instructor before you start the course.

If You Are Exposed to Blood or Body Fluids

If blood or other body fluids touch your skin, mouth, or eyes do the following:

Step	Action
1	If you are wearing gloves, take them off. (See "How to Take Off Protective Gloves.")
2	Immediately wash your hands and the contact area very well with soap and water. If the victim's body fluids have splattered in your eyes, nose, or the inside of your mouth, rinse these areas with lots of water.
3	Work up a soap lather for at least 15 seconds, and rinse your hands very well.
4	Dry your hands with a paper towel and use that paper towel to turn the faucet off.
5	Use waterless hand sanitizers *if you do not have immediate access to soap and water*. Wash your hands with soap and water as soon as you can.
6	Tell your company's emergency response program supervisor what happened as soon as possible. Then contact your healthcare professional.

FYI: Germs and Disease

Blood-borne diseases are diseases caused by germs in the victim's blood or other body fluids. A rescuer may catch a disease if germs in a victim's blood or body fluids enter the rescuer's body. The germs can enter through the rescuer's mouth or eyes or through a cut on the skin. To be safe, rescuers should wear personal protective equipment—gloves and eye shields (goggles)—to keep from touching the victim's blood or body fluids.

The most important blood-borne diseases are

- Human immunodeficiency virus (HIV), the virus that causes AIDS
- Hepatitis

How to Take Off Protective Gloves

When you give first aid, the outside of your gloves may touch blood or other body fluids. Take your gloves off without touching the outside of the gloves with your bare hands. Follow these steps to take off your gloves:

Step	Action
1	Grip one glove on the *outside* of the glove near the cuff and peel it down until it comes off inside out (Figure 6A).
2	Cup it with your other (gloved) hand (Figure 6B).
3	Place 2 fingers of your bare hand *inside* the cuff of the glove that is still on your hand (Figure 6C).
4	Peel that glove off so that it comes off "inside out" with the first glove inside it (Figure 6D).
5	If there is blood on the gloves, dispose of the gloves properly. • Put them in a biohazard waste bag if required to do so by your workplace (Figure 4). • If you do not have a biohazard waste bag, put the gloves in a plastic bag that can be sealed before you dispose of it.
6	Wash your hands after you give first aid so that you don't spread germs. Use waterless hand sanitizers *if you do not have immediate access to soap and water*. Wash your hands with soap and water as soon as you can.

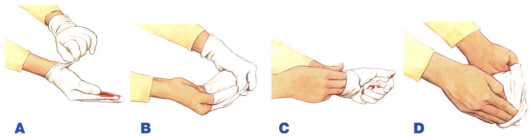

A **B** **C** **D**

Figure 6. Proper removal of protective gloves. Take your gloves off without touching the outside of the gloves with your bare hands.

Phoning for Help

The AHA Chain of Survival

The American Heart Association adult Chain of Survival (Figure 7) shows the most important actions needed to treat life-threatening emergencies in adults. The first link in this adult Chain of Survival is to recognize the emergency and activate the emergency response system. This section will teach you how and when to phone.

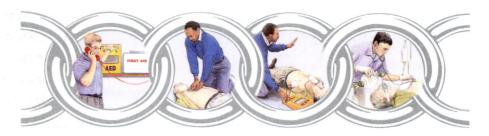

Figure 7. The AHA adult Chain of Survival. The 4 links or actions in the chain are (1) early recognition of the emergency and activation of the emergency response system, (2) early CPR, (3) early defibrillation, and (4) early advanced care.

What You Will Learn

By the end of this section you should be able to

- Tell how to phone your company's emergency response number (or 911)
- Tell how to contact the EMS system in your area
- Give examples of when you should phone your company's emergency response number (or 911) for help

Emergency Response Plan

Every place of business should have an emergency response plan. The emergency response plan tells workers *who, how,* and sometimes *when* to phone for help in an emergency.

How to Phone for Help

Your company's emergency response plan may be to call security, a response team, or the local EMS system number (in many communities this is 911). Make sure you know your phone system. Do you need to dial 9 to get an outside line before you dial your emergency response number (or 911)? You should know your company's emergency response number and phone that number whenever you need help.

Write the emergency response number in the box below, in the first aid kit, and on a large sign near the telephone (Figure 8).

In many communities you can contact EMS by phoning 911. Find out what the EMS number is in your community. If you don't know the number, phone "0" (operator). Some companies have emergency call buttons. If that button serves as the emergency response signal, you should know where it is located so that you can use it in an emergency.

> ### *Your Emergency Response Number*
>
> If there is an emergency in this area, phone _____ (fill in the blank).

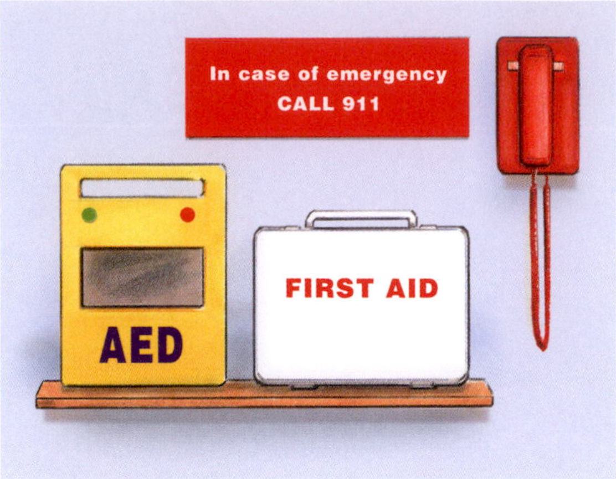

Figure 8. Write the emergency response phone number in the first aid kit and on a large sign near the telephone.

When to Phone for Help

Your company may have some instructions about when you should phone the emergency response number. In this student workbook we will tell you when to phone for help in specific emergencies. As a general rule, you should phone the emergency response number (or 911) and ask for help whenever

- Someone is seriously ill or hurt
- You are not sure what to do in an emergency

Remember: It is better to phone for help even if you might not need it than not to phone when someone does need help.

How to Phone for Help

The following table shows how to phone for help:

If you are	Then you should
Alone	• Yell for help while you start to check the victim. • If no one answers your yell and immediate care isn't needed — Leave the victim for a moment while you phone your emergency response number (or 911). — Get the first aid kit and automated external defibrillator (AED) if available. • Return to the victim.
With others	• Stay with the victim and be ready to give first aid or start the steps of CPR if you know how. • Send someone else to phone your emergency response number (or 911) and get the first aid kit and AED if available.

Answering Dispatcher Questions

When you phone your company's emergency response number (or 911), be prepared to answer some questions about the emergency. Here are some sample questions that an emergency response dispatcher may ask you:

- "Where is your emergency and what number are you calling from?"
- "What is the emergency?"
- "What is your name?"
- "Is the victim conscious?"
- "Is the victim breathing normally?"
- "Are you able to assist with CPR?"
- "Do you have access to an AED?"

Do not hang up until the dispatcher tells you to do so.

> **FYI: Emergency Dispatchers**
>
> When you phone for help, the emergency dispatcher may be able to tell you how to give first aid, do CPR, or use an AED.

If You Are in Doubt, Phone the Emergency Response Number

When in doubt, phone your company's emergency response number (or 911).

When to Phone Your Company's Emergency Response Number (or 911)

Phone your company's emergency response number (or 911) whenever someone is seriously ill or injured or when you are not sure what to do. Some examples include when a victim

- Does not respond to voice or touch
- Has chest pain or chest discomfort
- Has signs of stroke
- Has a problem breathing
- Has a severe injury or burn
- Has a seizure
- Suddenly can't move a part of the body
- Has received an electric shock
- Has been exposed to poison
- Tries to commit suicide or is assaulted, regardless of the victim's condition

Case Example (continued)

At the beginning of the second part of this section, you read a short case example:

A truck has struck an employee in the parking lot. You see a man lying on the ground. Several co-workers have gathered around him. You note that traffic is moving slowly around the crash.

You read the following question: Would you know what to do?

Now you know what to do.

As you approach the victim, you quickly look around to see who is there and if the scene is safe for you and the victim. You tell one worker to stand in the road and direct all traffic away from the scene. You ask another worker to phone your company's emergency response number (or 911) and get the first aid kit.

You kneel beside the victim. He is breathing and responds to you. You say, "Hi, my name is Joe/Jane Smith, and I have training in first aid. We've phoned for help. May I help you?" If the victim agrees, you can provide first aid. The first aid kit arrives, and as you put on protective gloves, you note that the victim's leg is bleeding.

If the victim does not agree, you stay with the victim until trained help arrives and takes over.

Finding the Problem

What You Will Learn

By the end of this section you should be able to show how to find out what the problem is when a victim is sick or hurt.

Overview

You must find out if the victim is injured or ill. This is the first step when you give first aid.

How to Find Out What the Problem Is

After you check the scene to be sure it is safe, you must find out what the problem is before you give first aid. Learn to look for problems in order of importance. First look for problems that may be life-threatening. Then look for other problems.

Steps to Find the Problem

The following steps will help you find out what the problem is. They are listed in order of importance, with the most important step listed first.

Step	Action
1	When you arrive at the scene, check the scene to be sure it is safe. As you walk toward the victim, try to **look for signs of the cause of the problem.**
2	Check whether the victim responds. **Tap the victim and shout, "Are you OK?"** (Figure 9). • A victim who "responds" will react in some way to your voice or touch. But remember that a victim who responds now may stop responding, so you have to keep rechecking. — A victim who responds and is awake may be able to answer your questions. Tell the victim you are there to help, ask permission to help, and ask what the problem is. — A victim may only be able to move or just moan or groan when you tap him and shout. If so, phone or send someone to phone your emergency response number (or 911) and get the first aid kit. • A victim who "does not respond" does not move or react in any way when you tap him and shout. Phone or send someone to phone your emergency response number (or 911) and get the first aid kit and AED.
3	**Next, open the airway with a head tilt-chin lift (Figure 10).** • If a victim responds and is awake, the victim is breathing. You will not need to open the airway. • If the victim does not respond or only moves or moans or groans, you have to open the airway before you can check if the victim is breathing: — Tilt the head by pushing back on the forehead. — Lift the chin by putting your fingers on the bony part of the chin. Do not press the soft tissues of the neck or under the chin. — Lift the chin to move the jaw forward.
4	**Check whether the victim is breathing.** • Place your ear next to the victim's mouth and nose. • **Look** to see whether the chest is moving. • **Listen** for breaths. • **Feel** for breaths on your cheek.
5	**Next, look for any obvious signs of injury, such as bleeding, broken bones, burns, or bites.** (You will learn about each of these problems later.)
6	**Finally, look for medical information jewelry** (Figure 11). This tells you if the victim has a serious medical condition.

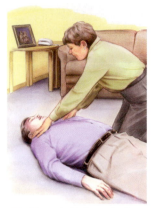

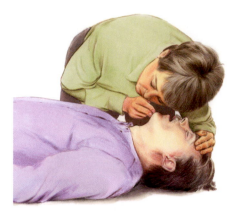

Figure 9. Check if the victim responds. Tap the victim and shout, "Are you OK?"

Figure 10. Open the airway with a head tilt–chin lift.

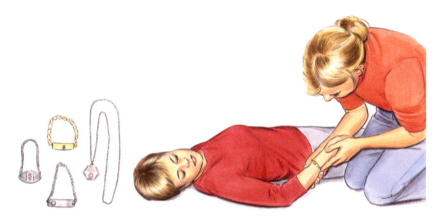

Figure 11. Look for medical information jewelry.

FYI: Airway Obstruction in the Victim Who Does Not Respond

The muscles at the back of the throat relax in a victim who does not respond. When the muscles relax, the tongue may fall back and block the airway. A victim with a blocked airway cannot breathe.

Tilting the head back and lifting the chin forward (Figure 10) pulls the tongue away from the back of the throat and opens the airway. You have to open the airway in a victim who does not respond before you can check whether the victim is breathing. You may have to open the airway in a victim who responds only by moaning or groaning.

Case Example

You are giving first aid to a victim when trained help arrives and takes over. You tell them what happened. They bring out a lot of equipment and work to save the victim. You stand on the side. Trained help places the victim in an ambulance and drives away. As you fill out the forms required by your company, you begin to feel sad. The next day you find out that the victim is seriously injured. You become anxious and can't get the emergency out of your mind. You constantly wonder whether you could have done something more.

What You Will Learn

By the end of this section you should be able to

- Tell how a first aid rescuer might feel after an emergency
- Explain your role in keeping first aid care confidential
- Tell which forms your company wants you to fill out after you give first aid

Medical Care for the Victim

As a first aid rescuer, you do not need to decide whether the victim needs medical care after you have given first aid. The victim, workplace policy, or EMS rescuers in consultation with the victim will make that decision.

Emotions of the Rescuer

After the excitement of an emergency you may feel a "letdown" even if the outcome is good. After all, during the initial moments of the crisis you had a lot of responsibility.

As soon as others, such as trained help, take over, you may feel pushed aside, left out, and unappreciated. You may feel guilty and blame yourself if the outcome is not good.

These feelings are common to all rescuers, no matter how experienced or knowledgeable they are. It is very important for you to be able to discuss your feelings with a counselor, doctor, nurse, or other healthcare provider.

Confidentiality

As a first aid rescuer you will learn private things about your co-workers, such as their medical condition. You ***must*** give all information about a victim to EMS rescuers and your company's emergency response program supervisor, but you must **not** share this information with other co-workers. Keep private things private (Figure 12).

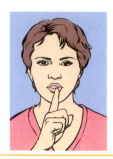

Figure 12. You must not share the victim's private medical information with other co-workers.

Reporting

Your company may ask you to fill out a report after you have given first aid. If your company does not have a special report form, you might want to complete a form similar to the one on page 20. Ask your supervisor if the form in this student workbook will meet your company's policy.

Appendix—Sample First Aid Kit

Item	Minimum Size or Volume	Quantity per package	Unit package size
List of important local emergency telephone numbers, including police, fire department, EMS, and poison control center			
Absorbent compress*	32 sq. in.	1	1
Adhesive bandage*	1″ × 3″	16	1
Adhesive tape*	5 yd. (total)	1 or 2	1 or 2
Antibiotic treatment*	1/32 oz.	6	1
Antiseptic swab*	0.14 fl. oz.	10	1
Antiseptic wipe*	1″ × 1″	10	1
Antiseptic towelette*	24 sq. in.	10	1
Bandage compress (2 in.)*	2″ × 36″	4	1
Bandage compress (3 in.)*	3″ × 60″	2	1
Bandage compress (4 in.)*	4″ × 72″	1	1
Burn dressing*	4″ × 4″	1	1 or 2
Burn treatment*†	1/32 oz.	6	1
CPR barrier*		1	1 or 2
Cold pack (4″ × 5″)*	4″ × 5″	1	2
Eye covering, with means of attachment*	2.9 sq. in.	2	1
Eye wash*	1 fl. oz. total	1	2

Item	Minimum Size or Volume	Quantity per package	Unit package size
Eye wash and covering, with means of attachment (1 fl. oz. total, 2.9 sq. in.)*	1 fl. oz. total 2.9 sq. in.	1 2	2
Gloves*		2 pair	1 or 2
Roller bandage (4 in.)*	4″ × 6 yd.	1	1
Roller bandage (2 in.)*	2″ × 6 yd.	1	1
Sterile pad*	3″ × 3″	2	1
Triangular bandage*	40″ × 40″ × 56″	4	1
Heartsaver First Aid Quick Reference Guide			

*Items meet the ANSI Z308.1-2003 standard.

†**Do not** put ointment on a burn unless a healthcare provider tells you to do so.

Date and time of report _____ Date and time of incident _____

Name of victim _____

Victim's employee no. _____ Location of emergency _____

Equipment involved in emergency _____

What was the victim's problem? _____

_____

Did the injury or illness involve any of the following? (Check all that apply.)

❏ CPR

❏ Automated external defibrillation (use of an AED)

❏ Head

❏ Breathing assistance

❏ Bleeding

❏ A fall

❏ An electric shock

❏ Burn

❏ Poisoning

❏ Eye (R) (L)

❏ Arm (R) (L)

❏ Leg (R) (L)

❏ Hand (R) (L)

❏ Foot (R) (L)

❏ Other _____

_____

_____

What happened?

_____

_____

_____

_____

List all responders who helped with the emergency:

_____

_____

_____

What happened to the victim? _____

Name of person completing report _____

Date _____

Question	Your Notes
1. *Fill in the blank with the correct word or words.* Personal protective equipment includes _____ to protect your hands from blood and other body fluids.	
2. *True or false* After you give first aid, you should wash your hands to help prevent illness. Circle your answer: True False	
3. *Fill in the blank with the correct word or words.* After you give first aid, you should put your used gloves in a _____ bag if one is available.	
4. *True or false* After you check the scene to be sure it is safe, you should first look for problems that may be life-threatening. Circle your answer: True False	

Medical Emergencies

Breathing Problems

What You Will Learn

By the end of this section you should be able to

- List the signs of a victim with a breathing problem
- Tell what to do when a victim has a breathing problem
- Show how to relieve choking
- List the signs and actions for a victim with a bad allergic reaction
- Show how to use an epinephrine pen

Breathing Problems

Body cells need oxygen to work properly. When you breathe, air goes down the air passages into the lungs. Oxygen then passes into the blood, which carries it to cells throughout the body. A person can't live without breathing.

A victim may develop a mild or severe block of the air passages by

- Something, such as food or a small object, going down "the wrong way" (into the air passages instead of the stomach)
- Swelling of the lining of the airway, for example, in a bad allergic reaction or severe asthma
- Infection
- Injuries to the head, neck, or chest

Breathing problems can also occur in victims with heart attacks, stroke, and some injuries.

Signs of Breathing Problems

You can tell if someone is having trouble breathing if the person

- Is breathing very fast or very slowly
- Is having trouble with every breath
- Has noisy breathing—you hear a sound or whistle as the air enters or leaves the lungs
- Doesn't have enough breath to make sounds or speak more than a few words at a time in between breaths, although the person is trying to say more

Many people with medical conditions, such as asthma, know about their condition and carry inhaler medicine that can make them feel better within minutes of using it (Figure 13).

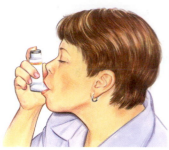

Figure 13. Many people with breathing problems carry inhaler medicines that can make them feel better within minutes.

Actions for Breathing Problems

Follow these steps for someone who is having trouble breathing:

Step	Action
1	Ask if the victim has medicine and help get it.
2	Phone the company emergency response number (or 911) if • The victim has no medicine • The victim does not get better after using his or her medicine • The victim's breathing gets worse, the victim has trouble speaking, or the victim stops responding
3	Be prepared to start the steps of CPR if the victim stops breathing.
4	Stay with the victim until trained help arrives and takes over.

Choking

Case Example

You are eating lunch in the cafeteria. You hear loud voices at the next table. A man is grabbing his throat and is unable to breathe, speak, or make any sounds. He looks very frightened. Several people are shouting at him. They don't know what to do.

Would you know what to do?

Signs and Actions for Choking

When food or another object gets in the airway, it can block the airway. Adults and children can easily choke while eating. Children can also easily choke when playing with small toys.

Choking can be a frightening emergency. If the block in the airway is severe, you must act quickly to remove the block. If you do, you can help the victim breathe.

Use the following table to know whether a victim is choking:

If the victim	Then the block in the airway is	And you should
• Can make sounds • Can cough loudly	Mild	• Stand by and let the victim cough • If you are worried about the victim's breathing, *phone your emergency response number (or 911)*
• Cannot breathe • Has a cough that is very quiet or has no sound • Cannot talk or make a sound • Cannot cry (younger child) • Has high-pitched, noisy breathing • Has bluish lips or skin • Makes the choking sign	Severe	• Act quickly • Follow the steps below

FYI: The Choking Sign

If someone is choking, he might use the choking sign (holding the neck with one or both hands) (Figure 14).

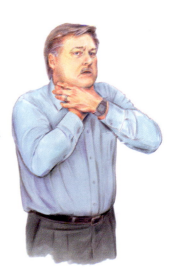

Figure 14. The choking sign. The victim holds his neck with one or both hands.

How to Help a Choking Person Over 1 Year of Age

When a victim is choking and suddenly cannot breathe, talk, or make any sounds, give abdominal thrusts. These thrusts are sometimes called the Heimlich maneuver. Abdominal thrusts push air from the lungs like a cough. This can help remove an object blocking the airway. You should give abdominal thrusts until the object is forced out and the victim can breathe, cough, or talk or until the victim stops responding.

Follow these steps to help a choking person who is 1 year of age and older:

Step	Action
1	If you think someone is choking, ask, "Are you choking?" If he nods, tell him you are going to help.
2	Kneel or stand firmly behind him and wrap your arms around him so that your hands are in front.
3	Make a fist with one hand.
4	Put the thumb side of your fist slightly above his navel (belly button) and well below the breastbone.
5	Grasp the fist with your other hand and give quick upward thrusts into his abdomen (Figure 15).
6	Give thrusts until the object is forced out and he can breathe, cough, or talk or until he stops responding.

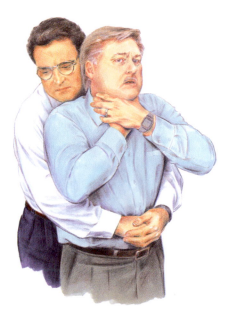

Figure 15. Give upward thrusts into the victim's abdomen.

Actions for a Choking Victim Who Stops Responding

If you cannot remove the object, the victim will stop responding. When the victim stops responding, follow these steps:

Step	Action
1	Yell for help. If someone comes, send that person to phone your emergency response number (or 911) and get the AED if available.
2	Lower the victim to the ground, face up. • If you are alone with the adult victim, phone your emergency response number (or 911) and get the AED. Then return to the victim and start the steps of CPR if you know how. (See Adult CPR on page 91.) • If you are alone with the child victim, start the steps of CPR if you know how. (See Child CPR on page 98.)
3	Every time you open the airway to give breaths, open the victim's mouth wide and look for the object (Figure 16). If you see an object, remove it with your fingers. If you do not see an object, keep giving sets of 30 compressions and 2 breaths until an AED arrives, the victim starts to move, or trained help arrives and takes over.
4	After about 5 cycles or 2 minutes, if you are alone, leave the child victim to call your emergency response number (or 911) and get the AED if available.
5	Return to the child victim and continue the steps of CPR if you know how.

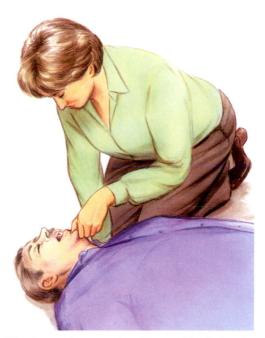

Figure 16. Open the mouth wide and look for the object.

FYI: Asking a Victim About Choking

Sometimes a victim is too young to answer your question or cannot answer your question for some other reason.

If the adult or child victim does not respond or cannot answer and you think the victim is choking, give abdominal thrusts until the object is forced out and the victim can breathe, cough, or talk or until the victim stops responding.

Actions to Help a Choking Large Person or Pregnant Woman

If the choking victim is in the late stages of pregnancy or is very large, use chest thrusts instead of abdominal thrusts (Figure 17).

Follow the same steps as above except for where you place your arms and hands. Put your arms under the victim's armpits and your hands on the center of the victim's chest. Pull straight back to give the chest thrusts.

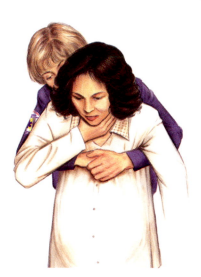

Figure 17. Chest thrusts on a choking large person or pregnant woman.

Case Example (continued)

At the beginning of this discussion, you read a Case Example:

You are eating lunch in the cafeteria. You hear loud voices at the next table. A man is grabbing his throat and is unable to breathe, speak, or make any sounds. He looks very frightened. Several people are shouting at him. They don't know what to do.

You read this question: Would you know what to do?

Now you know what to do.

You ask the victim, "Are you choking?" He nods. You say, "I'm going to help you." You stand behind him, wrap your arms around his abdomen, and give several abdominal thrusts. A piece of meat flies out of his mouth. Now he can talk and breathe more easily. He thanks you.

Bad Allergic Reactions

Case Example

At a company picnic a 38-year-old woman eats a cookie and complains that she is having trouble breathing. She tells you that she is very allergic to peanuts.

Would you know what to do?

Allergic Reactions

Many allergic reactions are *mild,* but you should remember that *a mild allergic reaction can become a bad allergic reaction within minutes.*

> **FYI: Common Allergies**
>
> People can be allergic to many things, including
> - Many foods, such as eggs, peanuts, chocolate
> - Insect stings or bites, especially bee stings

Signs of Mild and Bad Allergic Reactions

The following table shows signs of mild and bad allergic reactions:

Mild Allergic Reaction	Bad Allergic Reaction
• A stuffy nose, sneezing, and itching around the eyes • Itching of the skin • Raised, red rash on the skin (hives) (Figure 18)	• Trouble breathing • Swelling of the tongue and face • Fainting

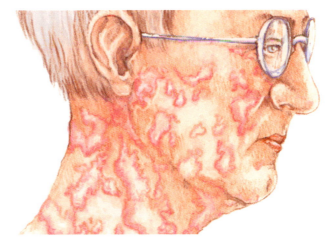

Figure 18. One sign of an allergic reaction can be a raised, red rash on the skin.

Actions for Bad Allergic Reactions

A bad allergic reaction can be life-threatening and is an emergency. Follow these steps if you see signs of a *bad* allergic reaction:

Step	Action
1	Make sure the scene is safe.
2	Phone or send someone to phone your company's emergency response number (or 911) and get the first aid kit.
3	If the victim responds and has an epinephrine pen, help the victim to get it and ask the victim to use it. (An epinephrine pen is also called an epinephrine injector.) Victims who carry epinephrine pens should know when and how to use them. If the victim cannot give the injection, you may help if you are trained and approved to do so by your state regulations and by your company (see below).
4	If the victim stops responding, start the steps of CPR if you know how (see section on CPR).
5	If possible, save a sample of what caused the reaction. This may be helpful if this is the victim's first allergic reaction.

Using an Epinephrine Pen

Some states and organizations permit first aid rescuers to help people use their epinephrine pen (see "How to Use an Epinephrine Pen").

An epinephrine pen is also called an epinephrine injector. It contains a small dose of medicine that can be injected through clothing (the side of the victim's leg). It will help someone with a bad allergic reaction breathe more easily. It usually takes several minutes before the medicine in the epinephrine pen starts to work.

Case Example (continued)

At the beginning of this discussion about Allergic Reactions, you read the following Case Example:

At a company picnic a 38-year-old woman eats a cookie and complains that she is having trouble breathing. She tells you that she is very allergic to peanuts.

You read this question: Would you know what to do?

Now you know what to do.

You ask a co-worker to phone your company's emergency response number (or 911) and get the first aid kit. You introduce yourself and offer to help. The woman lets you help her. You note that the victim is having trouble breathing. She is making high-pitched, noisy breathing sounds. Her tongue and face are starting to swell. She tells you that she has an epinephrine pen in her purse. You remove the epinephrine pen from the victim's purse and help her use it.

How to Use an Epinephrine Pen

The epinephrine injection is given in the side of the thigh.

Follow these steps to use an epinephrine pen:

Step	Action
1	Get the prescribed epinephrine pen.
2	Take off the safety cap (Figure 19A). Follow the instructions printed on the package.
3	Hold the epinephrine pen in your fist without touching either end because the needle comes out of one end.
4	Press the tip of the pen hard against the side of the victim's thigh, about halfway between the hip and knee (Figure 19B). You can give the epinephrine pen directly to the skin or through clothing.
5	Hold the pen in place for several seconds. Some of the medication will remain in the pen after you use it.
6	Rub the injection spot for several seconds.
7	After using the epinephrine pen, follow your organization's policy for "sharps" disposal or give the pen to the trained help for proper disposal.
8	Write down the time of the injection. This information is important for the victim's care by trained help. You can write it on a piece of paper and later transfer the time of the injection to your report.
9	Stay with the victim until trained help arrives and takes over.

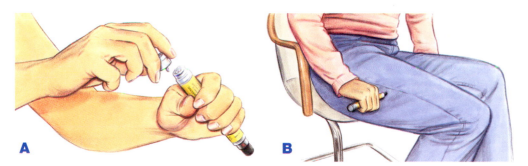

Figure 19. Using an epinephrine pen. **A.** Take off the safety cap. **B.** Press the tip of the pen hard against the side of the victim's thigh.

Heart Attack

Case Example

A middle-aged co-worker complains that he has an uncomfortable pressure in his chest that has been present for the last 5 minutes. You introduce yourself and ask if you may help. You notice that he is short of breath.

Would you know what to do?

What You Will Learn

By the end of this section you should be able to

- List several words that a victim may use to describe discomfort, pain, or pressure caused by a heart attack
- Describe where the pain or pressure of a heart attack might be located
- Describe first aid actions for a victim with chest discomfort, pain, or pressure

Signs of a Heart Attack

Signs of a heart attack may include

- **Chest discomfort.** Most heart attacks involve discomfort in the center of the chest that lasts more than a few minutes or that goes away and comes back. It can feel like uncomfortable pressure, squeezing, fullness, or pain (Figure 20).
- **Discomfort in other areas of the upper body.** Symptoms can include pain or discomfort in one or both arms, the back, neck, jaw, or stomach.
- **Shortness of breath.** May occur with or without chest discomfort.
- **Other signs** may include cold sweat, nausea, or lightheadedness.

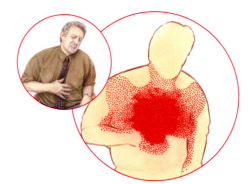

Figure 20. Typical locations of pain caused by a heart attack.

Signs of Heart Attack in Women, the Elderly, and People With Diabetes

Signs of a heart attack are often less clear in women, the elderly, and people with diabetes. These people may describe the uncomfortable feeling in the chest as an ache, heartburn, or indigestion, or the uncomfortable feeling may be in the back, jaw, neck, or shoulder. They may also complain of shortness of breath or have nausea or vomiting.

If You Suspect a Heart Attack, Phone the Emergency Response Number

A person having a heart attack is usually awake and can talk but may have an uncomfortable feeling, such as pain or pressure, in the chest or other signs of a heart attack. The first minutes of a heart attack are the most important because that is when the victim is likely to get worse and may die. These first minutes are also important because many of the treatments for heart attack will be most successful if they are given soon after the onset of signs of the heart attack. If you think that someone may be having a heart attack, phone your company's emergency response number (or 911) right away. Minutes count!

Actions for Heart Attack

Many people with an uncomfortable feeling in the chest will not admit that it may be caused by a heart attack. People often say, "I'm too healthy," "I don't want to bother the doctor," "I don't want to frighten my wife," or "I'll feel silly if it isn't a heart attack." If the victim does not act, *you—the rescuer—*must act.

Follow these steps if someone has any of the signs of a possible heart attack:

Step	Action
1	Have the victim sit quietly.
2	Phone or have someone phone your company's emergency response number (or 911).
3	Ask someone to get the first aid kit and AED if available.
4	Be ready to start the steps of CPR and use the AED if the victim stops responding.

Case Example (continued)

At the beginning of this section, you read this Case Example:

A middle-aged co-worker complains of an uncomfortable feeling of pressure in his chest, which he has had for the last 5 minutes. You introduce yourself and ask if you may help. He says, "Yes." You notice that he is short of breath.

You read this question: Would you know what to do?

Now you know what to do.

You ask your co-worker to sit quietly while you phone your company's emergency response number (or 911). He says, "Don't bother anyone. It's probably just something I ate." You ignore him and continue to phone.

FYI: Sudden Cardiac Arrest

Heart disease is the single biggest cause of death in the United States. Each year about 330,000 people die outside of hospitals or in Emergency Departments when the heart suddenly stops beating **(sudden cardiac arrest).**

Sudden cardiac arrest after a heart attack is most likely during the *first 4 hours* after the signs of a heart attack begin. So it is important that you phone the emergency response number (or 911) as soon as you suspect that someone is having a heart attack.

A person having a heart attack is less likely to die if you start the American Heart Association Chain of Survival immediately by phoning for help and being prepared to start the steps of CPR and use an AED (discussed later in this book).

Fainting

Case Example

A co-worker is squatting in front of the bottom shelf, looking for equipment. He stands up suddenly, grabs some boxes, and then falls to the ground. As you walk toward him, you see that his eyes are closed and he is not moving. By the time you get to him, he opens his eyes, starts moving, and says, "I'm OK."

Would you know what to do?

What You Will Learn

By the end of this section you should be able to

- Describe what fainting is
- Describe the first aid actions for fainting

Signs of Fainting

Fainting is a short period when a person stops responding for less than a minute and then seems fine. Seconds before the victim stops responding, he feels dizzy.

Fainting often occurs when the victim

- Stands without moving for a long time, especially if it is hot
- Suddenly stands after squatting or bending down
- Receives bad news

Actions for Fainting

Follow these steps if a person is dizzy but still responds:

Step	Action
1	Make sure the scene is safe.
2	Help the victim lie flat on the floor.

If a person faints and then starts to respond:

Step	Action
1	Ask the victim to continue to lie flat on the floor until all dizziness goes away.
2	If the victim remains dizzy, raise the victim's legs just above the level of the heart and keep them elevated until the victim is no longer dizzy.
3	If the victim fell, look for injuries caused by the victim's fall.
4	Once the victim is no longer dizzy, help the victim to sit up very slowly and briefly remain sitting before slowly standing.

Case Example (continued)

At the beginning of this section, you read the following Case Example:

A co-worker is squatting in front of the bottom shelf, looking for equipment. He stands up suddenly, grabs some boxes, and then falls to the ground. As you walk toward him, you see that his eyes are closed and he is not moving. By the time you get to him, he opens his eyes, starts moving and says, "I'm OK."

You read this question: Would you know what to do?

Now you know what to do.

You introduce yourself and ask if you may help. He agrees, and you ask the victim to continue to lie down. After a few minutes, you ask the victim if he is dizzy. When he tells you that he is not dizzy, you help him sit up slowly and then you help him to stand. After the victim sits up slowly and then stands up with your help, he says that he is fine and thanks you. You ask him to lie down again if he feels dizzy.

Diabetes and Low Blood Sugar

Case Example

Your team has worked without a lunch break and it is late afternoon. You notice that one of your team members has become very angry during the meeting. She is pale and sweating, although the room is not especially warm. She then looks tired and gets quieter. You ask if you may help. She tells you that she feels very sleepy. She says she has diabetes and probably should have eaten by now.

Would you know what to do?

What You Will Learn

By the end of this section you should be able to

- Tell the signs of low blood sugar in a person with diabetes
- List the first aid actions for low blood sugar in a person with diabetes

What Causes Low Blood Sugar

Insulin in the body helps turn sugar into energy. Since people with diabetes do not make enough insulin, they may give themselves insulin injections. If a person with diabetes doesn't eat enough sugar for the amount of insulin injected, the sugar level in the blood drops. Low blood sugar causes the victim's behavior to change.

Low Blood Sugar

Low blood sugar can occur if a person with diabetes

- Has not eaten or has vomited
- Has not eaten enough food for the level of activity and amount of insulin already in the bloodstream (such as exercise)
- Has injected too much insulin

Signs of Low Blood Sugar

Signs of low blood sugar can appear quickly and may include

- A change in behavior, such as confusion or irritability
- Sleepiness or even not responding
- Hunger, thirst, or weakness
- Sweating, pale skin color
- A seizure (see the section on seizures)

Actions for Low Blood Sugar

Follow these steps if the victim is *responding* and shows signs of low blood sugar:

Step	Action
1	If you think that the blood sugar is low and the victim can sit up and swallow, give the victim something containing sugar to eat or drink (see table below).
2	Have the victim sit quietly or lie down.
3	Phone or have someone phone your company's emergency response number (or 911) if the victim does not feel better within a few minutes after eating or drinking something containing sugar.

> **FYI: What to Give for Low Blood Sugar**
>
> The following shows what to give a victim with diabetes who has low blood sugar:
>
> - Fruit juice
> - Packet of sugar or honey
> - Non-diet soda
>
> Do **not** give foods that contain little or no sugar such as
>
> - Diet soda
> - Chocolate
> - Artificial sweetner

If the victim is unable to sit up or swallow or if the victim stops responding:

Step	Action
1	Phone or send someone to phone your company's emergency response number (or 911).
2	Do not give the victim anything to eat or drink. It may cause more harm.
3	If the victim is having a seizure, follow the steps in the section on seizures.
4	If the victim is not having a seizure and you do not suspect that the victim has a head, neck, or spine injury, roll the victim to his side to help keep the airway open.
5	Start the steps of CPR if you know how. (See "CPR and AED.")

Case Example (continued)

At the beginning of this section, you read the following Case Example:

Your team has worked without a lunch break and it is late afternoon. You notice that one of your team members has become very angry during the meeting. You also notice that she is pale and sweating, although the room is not especially warm. She then looks tired and gets quieter. You ask if you may help. She tells you that she feels very sleepy. She says she has diabetes and probably should have eaten by now.

You read this question: Would you know what to do?

Now you know what to do.

You look in the refrigerator in the lounge area for a drink that contains sugar. You do not pick a diet soda. You find some orange juice and bring it to her. She drinks it and soon feels much better. She thanks you for your help.

Stroke

Case Example

Your supervisor is talking to you. Suddenly he stops speaking, and then his right arm falls to his side. When he tries to speak, you notice that one side of his mouth is lower than the other side. After a few seconds you help him sit on the floor against the wall, but he is having trouble sitting upright.

Would you know what to do?

What You Will Learn

By the end of this section you should be able to

- List 3 signs of stroke
- Describe the first aid actions for stroke

Understanding Stroke

Strokes occur when blood stops flowing to a part of the brain. This can happen if there is bleeding in the brain or if a blood vessel in the brain becomes blocked. The signs of a stroke are usually very sudden.

It is important to recognize the signs of a stroke and get fast medical care because new treatments are now available. There are treatments that can decrease injury from a stroke and improve recovery, but these treatments must be given within the first hours after the first signs of stroke appear.

Signs of Stroke

The warning signs of stroke are

- Sudden numbness or weakness of the face, arm, or leg, especially on one side of the body
- Sudden confusion, trouble speaking or understanding
- Sudden trouble seeing in one or both eyes
- Sudden trouble walking, dizziness, loss of balance or coordination
- Sudden, severe headache with no known cause

Actions for Stroke

Follow these steps if you think someone is having a stroke

Step	Action
1	Make sure the scene is safe.
2	Phone or ask someone to phone your company's emergency response number (or 911) and get the first aid kit.
3	If the victim does not respond, start the steps of CPR if you know how (see section on CPR).

Case Example (continued)

At the beginning of this section, you read the following Case Example:

Your supervisor is talking to you. Suddenly he stops speaking, and then his right arm falls to his side. When he tries to speak, you notice that one side of his mouth is lower than the other side. After a few seconds you help him sit on the floor against the wall, but he is having trouble sitting upright.

You read this question: Would you know what to do?

Now you know what to do.

You ask if you may help. He nods and is breathing normally, but he can't speak and is unable to move his right arm, hand, or leg. He has no signs of injury. Since no one else is present, you leave to phone your company's emergency response number (or 911) and get the first aid kit. When you return, you continue to check his breathing until trained help arrives and takes over.

Seizures

Case Example

You are at work and hear a cry for help. You grab your first aid kit and run to see what the problem is. You find a co-worker on the ground surrounded by people. The man's body, arms, and legs are jerking.

Would you know what to do?

What You Will Learn

By the end of this section you should be able to

- Tell the signs of a seizure
- List the first aid actions for a person having a seizure

Some Causes of Seizures

A medical condition called epilepsy often causes seizures. But *not all* seizures are due to epilepsy. Seizures can also be caused by

- Head injury
- Low blood sugar
- Heat-related injury
- Poisons

Signs of a Seizure

During some types of seizures the victim may

- Lose muscle control
- Fall to the ground
- Have jerking movements of the arms and legs and sometimes other parts of the body
- Stop responding

Actions for a Seizure

Most seizures stop within a few minutes. During a seizure you should

Step	Action
1	Protect the victim from injury by • Moving furniture or other objects out of the victim's way • Placing a pad or towel under the victim's head
2	Phone or have someone phone your company's emergency response number (or 911).
3	After the seizure, check to see if the victim is breathing. If the victim does not respond, start the steps of CPR if you know how.
4	If you do not suspect that the victim has a head, neck, or spine injury, roll the victim to his side.
5	Stay with the victim until he starts responding.
6	If you have called your emergency response number (or 911), stay with the victim until trained help arrives and takes over.

After a seizure it is not unusual for the victim to be confused or to fall asleep.

Case Example (continued)

At the beginning of this section, you read the following Case Example:

You are at work and hear a cry for help. You grab your first aid kit and run to see what the problem is. You find a co-worker on the ground surrounded by people. The man's body, arms, and legs are jerking.

You read this question: Would you know what to do?

Now you know what to do.

You make sure that the area is safe for the victim. You ask everyone to step back, and you put a jacket under the victim's head. Within a few minutes the jerking movements stop. You check the victim's breathing. He is breathing normally. When you ask if he can hear you, he opens his eyes and nods. At first he is confused, but then he begins to respond normally.

Do Not

When giving first aid to a victim having a seizure

- Do not hold the victim down
- Do not put anything in the victim's mouth

The victim may bite his tongue during a seizure. You can give first aid for that injury after the seizure stops.

Shock

Case Example

You are giving first aid to a victim of a car crash. The victim complains of pain in her abdomen. You notice that she is becoming restless. Her skin is pale, cool, and moist. She says she is cold and complains of being sick to her stomach.

Would you know what to do?

What You Will Learn

By the end of this section you should be able to

- List the signs of shock
- List the first aid actions for shock

Understanding Shock

Shock develops when there is not enough blood flowing to the cells of the body. In adults shock is most often present if the victim

- Loses a lot of blood that you may or may not be able to see
- Has a severe heart attack
- Has a bad allergic reaction

Signs of Shock

A victim in shock may

- Feel weak, faint, or dizzy
- Have pale or grayish skin
- Act restless, agitated, or confused
- Be cold and clammy to the touch

Actions for Shock

Follow these steps when giving first aid to a victim showing signs of shock:

Step	Action
1	Make sure the scene is safe for you and the victim.
2	Phone or send someone to phone your company's emergency response number (or 911) and get the first aid kit.
3	Help the victim lie on her back.
4	If there is no leg injury or pain, raise the victim's legs just above the level of the heart (Figure 21).
5	Use pressure to stop bleeding that you can see. (See "Bleeding You Can See.")
6	Cover the victim to keep the victim warm (you can use a Mylar blanket if there is one in the first aid kit).

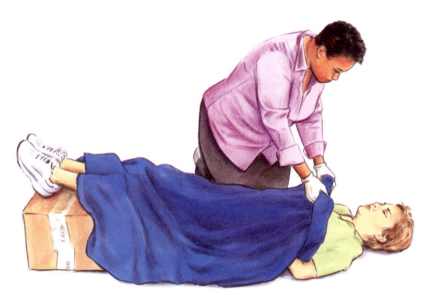

Figure 21. If there is no leg injury or pain, raise the victim's legs just above the level of the heart. Keep the victim warm with a blanket.

FYI: Raising a Victim's Legs

If a victim seems to be in shock, you may raise the victim's legs if it doesn't hurt the victim to do so. Do not raise the victim's legs if you know the victim has an injury or pain in the legs.

FYI: Understanding the Signs of Shock

When a victim loses a lot of blood or when the victim's blood does not circulate properly, there is not enough blood delivered to the cells of the body. We call this condition "shock."

In many forms of shock some blood is pumped to the most important organs of the body—the brain and heart—and less blood is pumped to the skin and muscles. The skin becomes cool, pale, and sweaty and the victim may vomit, feel thirsty, restless, weak, faint, or dizzy. The victim may stop responding.

Case Example (continued)

At the beginning of this section, you read the following Case Example:

You are giving first aid to a victim of a car crash. The victim complains of pain in her abdomen. You notice that she is becoming restless. Her skin is pale, cool, and moist. She says she is cold and complains of being sick to her stomach.

You read this question: Would you know what to do?

Now you know what to do.

You make sure that the scene is safe for you and the victim. You ask someone to direct traffic away from the scene. You ask another person to phone your company's emergency response number (or 911) and get the first aid kit. You decide that the victim has signs of shock. She is already lying on her back. She has no signs of a leg injury. You raise her legs just above the level of the heart by putting a box under them. You cover her with a Mylar blanket from the first aid kit. You keep looking to make sure she does not stop responding. Trained help arrives and takes over.

Question	Your Notes
1. *True or false* If an adult is eating and suddenly coughs and cannot breathe, talk, or make any sounds, you should ask if she is choking. If she nods, tell her you are going to help and give abdominal thrusts. Circle your answer: True False	
2. *True or false* When giving abdominal thrusts to an adult who is choking, you should put the thumb side of your fist slightly above her navel (belly button) and well below the breastbone. Circle your answer: True False	
3. *True or false* Signs of a bad allergic reaction include trouble breathing, swelling of the tongue and face, and fainting. Circle your answer: True False	
4. *Fill in the blank with the correct word or words.* A person having a _____ _____ may have an uncomfortable feeling, such as pain or pressure, in the chest or other areas of the body.	
5. *Fill in the blank with the correct word or words.* The warning signs of _____ include sudden numbness or weakness of the face, arm, or leg, especially on one side of the body.	
6. *True or false* If a victim with low blood sugar is responding and can sit up and swallow, you should give the victim something that contains sugar to eat or drink. Circle your answer: True False	
7. *True or false* If a victim is having a seizure, you should not put anything in his mouth. Circle your answer: True False	

Question	Your Notes
8. *True or false* When a victim is having a seizure, you should try to hold the victim down to protect the victim from injury. Circle your answer:　　True　　False	
9. *Fill in the blank with the correct word or words.* If a victim is showing signs of shock, you should help the victim lie on his back and raise his _____.	

Injury Emergencies

Bleeding You Can See

Case Example

A co-worker is hit by a car in front of your workplace. You make sure that your company's emergency response number (or 911) has been called. You get your first aid kit and run to help. You check the scene to make sure it is safe. You ask a bystander to stop traffic. The victim responds and complains of pain in her arm and stomach. You notice that her arm is bleeding.

Would you know what to do?

What You Will Learn

By the end of this section you should be able to

- List the first aid actions for bleeding that you can see
- Show how to stop bleeding

Bleeding You Can See

Bleeding is one of the most frightening emergencies. But many cuts are small and you can easily stop the bleeding. When a large blood vessel is cut or torn, the victim can lose a large amount of blood within minutes. That's why you have to act fast.

Remember:

- Remain calm.
- You can stop most bleeding with pressure.
- Bleeding often looks a lot worse than it is.

Actions for Bleeding You Can See

Take the following actions to stop bleeding that you can see:

Step	Action
1	Make sure that the scene is safe for you and the victim.
2	Send someone to get the first aid kit.
3	Wear personal protective equipment (gloves and eye protection if available).
4	If the victim is able, ask the victim to put pressure over the wound with a large clean dressing while you put on gloves and eye protection.

(continued)

Step	Action
5	You should be able to stop most bleeding with pressure alone. Put firm pressure on the dressing over the bleeding area with the flat part of your fingers or the palm of your hand (Figure 22). A small amount of pressure is all that you need to control bleeding from a scrape. You have to press harder to stop severe bleeding.
6	If the bleeding does not stop, add a second dressing and press harder (Figure 23). Do not remove the first dressing because it might pull off some blood clots and cause the wound to bleed more.
7	Check for signs of shock.
8	Phone or ask someone to phone your company's emergency response number (or 911) if • There is a lot of bleeding • You cannot stop the bleeding • You see signs of shock • The injury is from a fall and you suspect a head, neck, or spine injury • You are not sure what to do

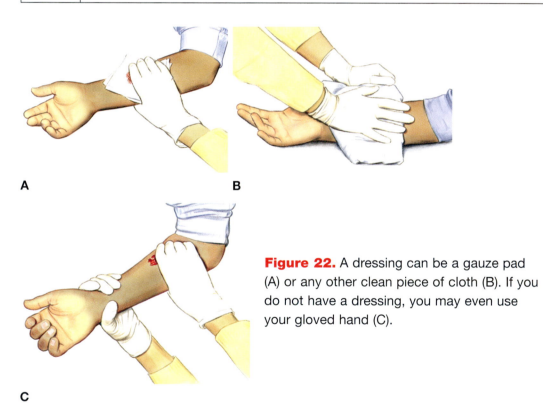

A

B

C

Figure 22. A dressing can be a gauze pad (A) or any other clean piece of cloth (B). If you do not have a dressing, you may even use your gloved hand (C).

FYI: Dressings

Use dressings to

- Stop bleeding with pressure
- Keep the wound clean

A dressing can be a gauze pad (Figure 22A) or any other clean piece of cloth (Figure 22B). Gauze pads come in different sizes. You should be able to find them in your first aid kit. Choose a size that covers the wound. Use sterile gauze pads on an open wound to lower the chance of infection. If you don't have a sterile dressing, use any clean cloth, such as a scarf or a shirt. You may even use your gloved hand (Figure 22C).

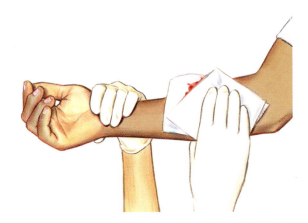

Figure 23. If a dressing becomes soaked with blood, add more dressings and press harder.

Actions for Minor Cuts and Scrapes

You can stop bleeding from minor cuts and scrapes using pressure. Follow these steps for minor cuts and scrapes:

Step	Action
1	Make sure the scene is safe for you and the victim.
2	Send someone to get the first aid kit.
3	Put on personal protective equipment.
4	Wash the wound well with water and soap if available.
5	Stop the bleeding with pressure.
6	Apply a dressing or bandage to the wound.

FYI: Antibiotic Creams

Wounds heal better and with less infection if an antibiotic ointment or cream is used. Triple antibiotic ointment appears to be better than single antibiotic ointment or cream.

Apply antibiotic ointment or cream only if the victim's wound is a small scrape or surface cut.

Actions for Major Cuts and Scrapes

Follow these steps if the cut or scrape is major and the victim is bleeding a lot:

Step	Action
1	Make sure the scene is safe for you and the victim.
2	Phone or send someone to phone your emergency response number (or 911) and get the first aid kit.
3	Put on personal protective equipment.
4	Stop any bleeding you can see using the skills you learned above.
5	Check for signs of shock.
6	Stay with the victim until trained help arrives and takes over.

Case Example (continued)

At the beginning of this section, you read the following Case Example:

A co-worker is hit by a car in front of your workplace. You make sure that your company's emergency response number (or 911) has been called. You get your first aid kit and run to help. You check the scene to make sure it is safe. You ask a bystander to stop traffic. The victim responds and complains of pain in her arm and stomach. You notice that her arm is bleeding.

You read this question: Would you know what to do?

Now you know what to do.

You identify yourself and offer to help. When the victim agrees, you check the victim and note that she is responding and bleeding from her right arm. You ask the victim to put pressure on the bleeding area of her arm while you put on protective gloves and an eye shield. You quickly put pressure on the bleeding area with your gloved hand. Then you apply firm pressure over a gauze pad that you get from the first aid kit. You look for signs of shock (see "Shock" on page 41).

Wounds

Overview

This section tells you how to give first aid for bleeding from

- Nose injuries
- Mouth injuries
- Puncturing objects
- Amputation

Bleeding From the Nose

With nosebleeds it can be hard to know how much bleeding there is because the victim often swallows some of the blood. This may cause the victim to vomit.

Actions for Bleeding From the Nose

Follow these steps when giving first aid to a victim with a nosebleed:

Step	Action
1	Make sure the scene is safe for you and the victim.
2	Send someone to get the first aid kit.
3	Put on personal protective equipment.
4	Press both sides of the victim's nostrils while the victim sits and leans *forward* (Figure 24).
5	Place constant pressure on both sides of the nostrils for a few minutes until the bleeding stops.
6	If bleeding continues, press harder.
7	Phone or ask someone to phone your company's emergency response number (or 911) if • You can't stop the bleeding in about 15 minutes • The bleeding is heavy, such as gushing blood • The victim has trouble breathing

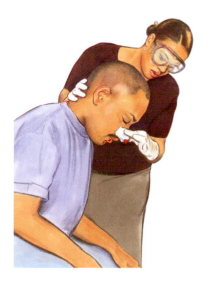

Figure 24. To stop a nosebleed, press both sides of the victim's nostrils while the victim sits and leans forward.

Do Not

When trying to stop a nosebleed

- *Do not* ask the victim to lean his head back.
- *Do not* use an icepack on the nose or forehead.
- *Do not* press on the bridge of the nose between the eyes (the upper bony part of the nose).

Bleeding From the Mouth

Like other bleeding you can see, you can usually stop bleeding from the mouth with pressure. But bleeding from the mouth can be serious if blood or broken teeth block the airway and cause breathing problems or if you can't reach the bleeding area.

Actions for Bleeding From the Mouth

Follow these steps when giving first aid to a victim with bleeding from the mouth:

Step	Action
1	Make sure that the scene is safe for you and the victim.
2	Send someone to get the first aid kit.
3	Put on personal protective equipment.
4	If the bleeding is from the tongue, lip, or cheek or another area you can easily reach, press the bleeding area with sterile gauze or a clean cloth (Figure 25).
5	If bleeding is deep in the mouth and you can't reach it easily, roll the victim to his side.
6	Check for signs of shock.
7	Watch the victim's breathing. Be ready to start the steps of CPR if needed and if you know how (see section on CPR).
8	Phone or ask someone to phone your company's emergency response number (or 911) if • You can't stop the bleeding • The victim has trouble breathing

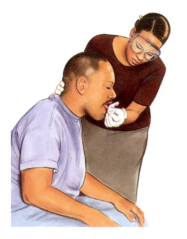

Figure 25. If the bleeding is from the tongue, lip, or cheek, press the bleeding area with sterile gauze or a clean cloth.

Injuries From Puncturing Objects

An object such as a knife or sharp stick can cause a penetrating injury or an injury that punctures the skin. It is important not to remove the object. Leave it in place until a healthcare provider can treat the injury.

Actions for Injuries From Puncturing Objects

Follow these steps when giving first aid to a victim with an injury from a puncturing object:

Step	Action
1	Make sure the scene is safe for you and the victim.
2	Phone or ask someone to phone your emergency response number (or 911) and get the first aid kit.
3	Put on personal protective equipment.
4	Stop any bleeding you can see.
5	Try to keep the victim from moving.
6	Check for signs of shock.

Do Not

If a person is injured and a sharp object, such as a nail or a knife, remains partly stuck in the body, *do not* take it out. Taking it out may cause more damage.

Amputations

If a part of the body, such as a finger, toe, hand, or foot is cut off (amputated), you should save the body part because doctors may be able to reattach it. You can preserve a detached body part at room temperature, but it will be in a better condition to be reattached if you keep it cool.

Actions for Amputation

Follow these steps when giving first aid to a victim with an amputation:

Step	Action
1	Make sure the scene is safe for you and the victim.
2	Phone or ask someone to phone your emergency response number (or 911) and get the first aid kit.
3	Put on personal protective equipment.
4	Stop the bleeding from the injured area with pressure. You will have to press for a long time with very firm pressure to stop the bleeding.
5	Look for signs of shock and give first aid as needed. (See "Actions for Shock" on page 42.)
6	If you find the amputated part, refer to "Protecting an Amputated Part" on the next page.
7	Stay with the victim until trained help arrives and takes over.

Protecting an Amputated Part

Follow these steps to protect an amputated part:

Step	Action
1	Rinse the amputated part with clean water (Figure 26A).
2	Cover or wrap the amputated part with a clean dressing.
3	If it will fit, place the amputated part in a watertight plastic bag (Figure 26B).
4	Place that bag in another container with ice or ice and water; label it with the victim's name, date, and time (Figure 26C).
5	Make sure it is sent to the hospital with the victim.

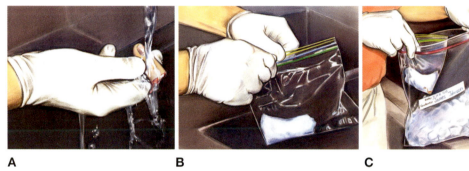

A   B   C

Figure 26. A, If you can find the amputated part, rinse it with sterile or clean water. Then cover or wrap it with a clean dressing. **B,** If it will fit, place it in a watertight plastic bag. **C,** Place that bag in another container with ice or ice and water; label it with the victim's name, date, and time; and make sure it is sent to the hospital with the victim.

> **Do Not**
>
> Never place the amputated body part directly on ice or in water because the ice or water may damage it.

Tooth Injuries

People with a mouth injury may have broken, loose, or knocked-out teeth. This can be a choking hazard.

Actions for Tooth Injuries

Follow these steps when giving first aid to a victim with a tooth injury:

Step	Action
1	Make sure the scene is safe for you and the victim.
2	Send someone to get the first aid kit.
3	Put on personal protective equipment.
4	Check the victim's mouth for any missing teeth, loose teeth, or parts of teeth.
5	If a tooth is loose, have the victim bite down on a piece of gauze to keep the tooth in place and call the victim's dentist.

Step	Action
6	If a tooth is chipped, gently clean the injured area and call the victim's dentist.
7	If the victim lost a tooth, rinse the tooth in water, put the tooth in a cup of milk, and immediately take the victim and tooth to a dentist or emergency department.
8	Apply pressure with gauze to stop any bleeding at the empty tooth socket.
9	Tell the victim to talk with a dentist if a tooth changes color after an injury.

Do Not

- *Do not* hold the tooth by the root. Hold the tooth by only the crown (the part of the tooth that does not go into the gums).
- *Do not* try to reinsert the tooth.

Bleeding You Can't See

What You Will Learn

By the end of this section you should be able to

- Tell when you should suspect bleeding inside the body
- List the first aid actions for bleeding you can't see

Bleeding You Can't See

A strong blow to the chest or abdomen or a fall can cause injury and bleeding inside the body. You may not see signs of this bleeding on the outside of the body at all, or you may see a bruise of the skin over the injured part of the body. An injury inside the body may be minor or severe.

When to Suspect Bleeding You Can't See

Suspect bleeding inside the body if a victim has

- An injury from a car crash, a pedestrian injury, or a fall from a height
- An injury to the abdomen or chest (including bruises such as seat belt marks)
- Sports injuries such as running into other people hard or being hit with a ball or bat
- Pain in the chest or abdomen after an injury
- Shortness of breath after an injury
- Coughed-up or vomited blood after an injury
- Signs of shock without bleeding that you can see
- A knife or gunshot wound

Actions for Bleeding You Can't See

Follow these steps when giving first aid to a victim who may have bleeding you can't see:

Step	Action
1	Make sure that the scene is safe for you and the victim.
2	Phone or ask someone to phone your company's emergency response number (or 911) and get the first aid kit and AED if available.
3	Have the victim lie down and keep still.
4	Check for signs of shock.
5	If the victim stops responding, start the steps of CPR if you know how (see section on CPR).

Case Example (continued)

In Case Examples earlier in "First Aid Basics" and this section, you read about a co-worker struck by a car:

A co-worker is hit by a car in front of your workplace. You make sure that your company's emergency response number (or 911) has been called. You get your first aid kit and run to help. You check the scene to make sure it is safe. You ask a bystander to stop traffic.

The victim responds and asks you to help. She complains of pain in her arm and stomach area. You stop the bleeding from the victim's arm and watch for signs of shock. The victim continues to complain of pain in the stomach area and becomes restless. Her skin is pale, cool, and moist. She is cold and sick to her stomach. Since she has no pain in the hip or leg, you raise her feet and rest them on a box. You cover her with a blanket. She continues to have pain in her stomach area.

You read the question: Would you know what to do?

Now you know what to do.

You think that the victim probably has bleeding inside the abdomen. You watch her closely to see if she keeps responding. You talk to her to keep her calm. You stay with her until trained help arrives and takes over.

Head, Neck, and Spine Injury

Case Example

A worker was unloading a truck when he was hit on the head by a forklift. When you arrive, he is lying on the ground. A crowd has gathered. You quickly look around. You note that the scene is safe for you and the victim. The forklift is not in the way, and there is no moving traffic. You ask someone to phone your company's emergency response number (or 911) and get the first aid kit. You ask another person to direct traffic away from the scene. You kneel by the victim's side and gently tap him and shout. He does not respond.

Would you know what to do?

What You Will Learn

By the end of this section you should be able to

- List signs of head, neck, and spine injury
- List first aid actions for a victim with a possible head, neck, and spine injury

When to Suspect a Head Injury

Suspect a head injury if the victim

- Fell from a height
- Was hit in the head
- Was injured while diving
- Was electrocuted
- Was involved in a car crash
- Was riding a bicycle or motorbike, was involved in a crash, and has no helmet or a broken helmet

Signs of Head Injury

You should suspect that a victim has a head injury if after an injury the victim

- Does not respond or only moves or moans or groans
- Is sleepy or confused
- Vomits
- Complains of a headache
- Has trouble seeing
- Has trouble walking or moving any part of the body
- Has a seizure

Neck and Spine Injuries

The bones of the spine protect the spinal cord. The spinal cord carries messages between the brain and the body.

If these bones are broken, the spinal cord may be injured. The victim may not be able to move his or her legs or arms and may lose feeling in parts of the body. Some people call this a "broken back."

When to Suspect a Neck or Spine Injury

Suspect that the spine bones are broken if a victim

- Has an injury to the upper part of the body, especially the head, back, or chest
- Was injured by a falling object or a forceful blow to the head or chest
- Was in a motor vehicle crash (in the vehicle or as a pedestrian)
- Fell from a height
- Was injured while under the influence of drugs or alcohol
- Had an injury that caused the victim to stop responding
- Is not fully alert
- Complains of neck or back pain, tingling in the arms or legs, or weakness
- Is injured while diving

Actions for Head, Neck, and Spine Injuries

Follow these steps when giving first aid to a victim with a possible head, neck, or spine injury:

Step	Action
1	Make sure that the scene is safe for you and the victim.
2	Phone or ask someone to phone your company's emergency response number (or 911) and get the first aid kit.
3	Hold the head and neck so that the head and neck do not move, bend, or twist (Figure 27).
4	Only turn or move the victim if • The victim is in danger • You need to do so to check breathing or open the victim's airway • The victim is vomiting
5	If the victim does not respond, start the steps of CPR if you know how.
6	If you must turn the victim, be sure to roll the victim while you support the victim's head, neck, and body in a straight line so that they do not twist, bend, or turn in any direction (Figure 28). This requires 2 rescuers.
7	If the victim responds but is vomiting, roll the victim onto her side.

Important

You may cause further injury to the spinal cord if you bend, twist, or turn the victim's head or neck. When you give first aid to a victim with a possible spine injury, you must not bend, twist, or turn the head or neck!

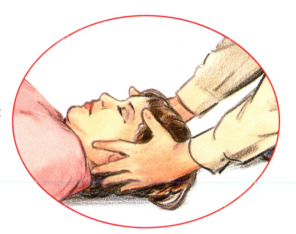

Figure 27. Hold the head and neck so that the neck does not move, bend, or twist.

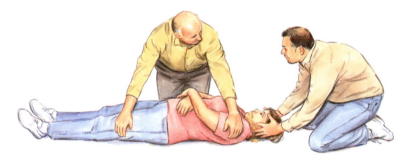

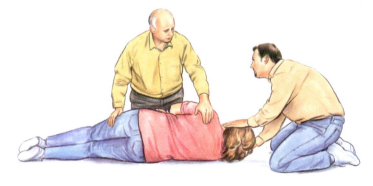

Figure 28. If you must turn the victim, be sure to roll the victim while you support the victim's head, neck, and body so that the head and neck are kept in line and do not twist, bend, or turn in any direction.

Case Example (continued)

At the beginning of this section, you read the following Case Example:

A worker was unloading a truck when he was hit on the head by a forklift. When you arrive, he is lying on the ground. A crowd has gathered. You quickly look around. You note that the scene is safe for you and the victim. The forklift is not in the way, and there is no moving traffic. You ask someone to phone your company's emergency response number (or 911) and get the first aid kit. You ask another person to direct traffic away from the scene. You kneel by the victim's side and gently tap him and shout. He does not respond.

You read this question: Would you know what to do?

Now you know what to do.

You hold the head and neck so the neck does not bend, twist, or move and you check the victim's breathing. He is breathing. When trained help arrives and takes over, you tell them what happened.

Broken Bones and Sprains

Case Example

While playing basketball, a co-worker falls and twists her ankle. When you arrive, she is sitting on the floor in pain. Her ankle is beginning to swell and is a bluish color.

Would you know what to do?

What You Will Learn

By the end of this section you should be able to list the first aid actions for broken bones and sprains

Understanding Bone, Joint, and Muscle Injuries

Injuries to bones, joints, and muscles are common. The injuries may include joint injuries, broken bones, and bruises (black-and-blue spots). Without an x-ray, it may be impossible to tell whether a bone is broken. But you will perform the same actions even if you don't know whether the bone is actually broken.

Joint Sprains

Joint sprains result from a twisting injury. The twisting injury causes tears in muscles and other structures around the joint. The tears cause pain. They may cause swelling and a blue color over the joint. Ice and rest decrease the amount of joint pain and swelling and help the joint to heal faster.

Actions for Broken Bones and Sprains

Follow these steps when giving first aid for a victim with a possible broken bone or sprain:

Step	Action
1	Make sure that the scene is safe for you and the victim.
2	Send someone to get the first aid kit. If you are alone, go get the first aid kit.
3	Put on personal protective equipment.
4	Check for signs of shock.
5	Don't try to straighten or move any injured part that is bent, deformed, or possibly broken (such as an arm, a leg, or a finger).
6	Cover any open wound with a clean dressing.
7	Put a plastic bag filled with ice on the injured area with a towel between the ice bag and the skin for up to 20 minutes (Figure 29).
8	Raise the injured body part if doing so does not cause the victim more pain.
9	Phone or ask someone to phone your emergency response number (or 911) if • There is a large open wound • The injured part is abnormally bent • You're not sure what to do
10	If it is painful, the victim should avoid using an injured body part until checked by a healthcare provider.

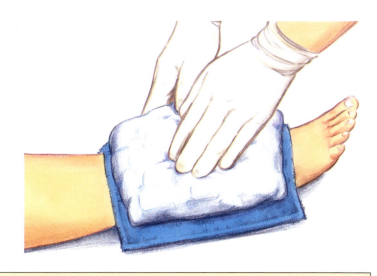

Figure 29. Put a plastic bag filled with ice on the injured area with a towel between the ice bag and the skin.

> ### *FYI: If Ice Is Not Available*
>
> You may use a cold pack, but it is not as cold and may not work as well as ice.

Case Example (continued)

At the beginning of this section about Broken Bones and Sprains, *you read this Case Example:*

While playing basketball, a co-worker falls and twists her ankle. When you arrive, she is sitting on the floor in pain. Her ankle is beginning to swell and is a bluish color.

You read this question: Would you know what to do?

Now you know what to do.

You introduce yourself and ask if you may help. When the victim agrees, you ask the victim to continue sitting on the floor. You ask someone to get the first aid kit. You ask a second person to get you some ice in a plastic bag. You put a towel on the ankle and put the ice bag on the towel. You hold the ice bag on the joint and take it off every 20 minutes. You raise the injured body part if doing so does not cause the victim more pain. You ask the victim to not walk on the foot until she is checked by a healthcare provider.

Burns and Electrocution

Causes of Burns

Burns are injuries that can be caused by contact with heat, electricity, or chemicals (see "Poison Emergencies" for information on chemical burns).

Case Example

A co-worker screams when she spills very hot coffee over her right hand and arm.

Would you know what to do?

What You Will Learn

By the end of this section you should be able to

- List the first aid actions for burns
- List the first aid actions for a victim of electrocution

Burns Caused by Heat

Heat burns can be caused by contact with fire, a hot surface, a hot liquid, or steam.

Actions for Small Burns

Follow these steps to give first aid to a victim with a small burn:

Step	Action
1	Make sure the scene is safe for you and the victim.
2	Send someone to get the first aid kit. If you are alone, go get the first aid kit.
3	If the burn area is small, cool it immediately with cold, but not ice cold, water (Figure 30).
4	You may cover the burn with a dry, nonstick sterile or clean dressing.
5	Phone or send someone to phone your emergency response number (or 911) if • There is a fire • The victim has a large burn • You are not sure what to do

Actions for Large Burns

Follow these steps to give first aid to a victim with a large burn:

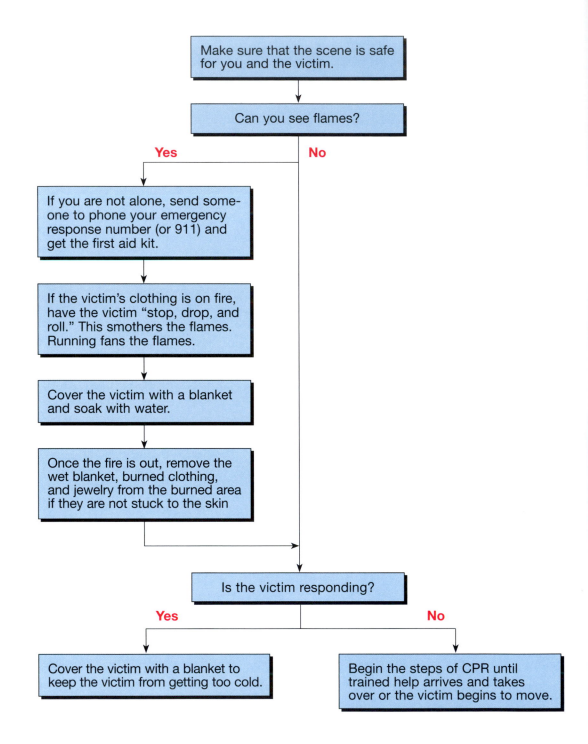

Make sure that the scene is safe for you and the victim.

Can you see flames?

Yes / **No**

If you are not alone, send someone to phone your emergency response number (or 911) and get the first aid kit.

If the victim's clothing is on fire, have the victim "stop, drop, and roll." This smothers the flames. Running fans the flames.

Cover the victim with a blanket and soak with water.

Once the fire is out, remove the wet blanket, burned clothing, and jewelry from the burned area if they are not stuck to the skin

Is the victim responding?

Yes / **No**

Cover the victim with a blanket to keep the victim from getting too cold.

Begin the steps of CPR until trained help arrives and takes over or the victim begins to move.

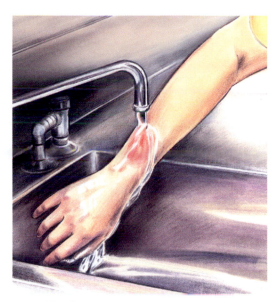

Figure 30. If possible, hold the burned area under cold running water.

Case Example (continued)

At the start of this section, you read this Case Example:

A co-worker screams when she spills very hot coffee over her right hand and arm.

You read this question: Would you know what to do?

Now you know what to do.

You introduce yourself and ask if you may help. When she agrees, you send someone to get the first aid kit. You roll up the co-worker's sleeve and see a red burned area. You ask the co-worker to put her hand and arm under cold running water and cool the burn. You then cover the burn with a clean, dry dressing.

Causes of Electrocution and Electrical Injuries

Electricity occurs naturally in the form of lightning or from manmade sources like an electrical current from an outlet or electrical wire. Electricity can cause burns on the surface and injure organs inside the body.

If electricity enters the body, it can cause severe damage. It can even cause the victim to stop breathing, or it can cause an abnormal heart rhythm that can be deadly. You may see marks or wounds where the electricity has entered and left the body. These marks may seem very small, but *you can't tell from the outside how much damage there is inside the body!*

Actions for Electrical Injury

Follow these steps for giving first aid for an electrical injury:

Step	Action
1	Make sure the scene is safe for you and the victim. Do not touch the victim as long as the victim is in contact with the power source. (See "FYI: Electrocution and Power Supplies" below.)
2	Phone or send someone to phone your company's emergency response number (or 911) and get an AED if available. (See "Using AEDs.")
3	When it is safe to touch the victim, check for a response. If the victim does not respond or stops responding, start the steps of CPR if you know how and use the AED if available. (See "CPR and AED.")
4	Check for signs of shock.
5	A healthcare provider should check all victims with an electrical injury.

FYI: Electrocution and Power Supplies

Do not touch the victim as long as the victim is in contact with the power source while the power is on. Electricity can travel from the source through the victim to you. It's best to turn off the main power switch (usually located near the fuse box).

If the electrocution is caused by *high voltage*, such as a fallen power line, immediately notify the proper authorities (phone your emergency response number or 911). Remember that if the voltage is high enough, it can travel through *everything* that touches the power line or source (even a wooden stick) and can hurt you. *Don't enter the area around the victim.* Don't try to pull away wires or other materials until the power has been turned off.

Do Not

When providing first aid for a burn

- *Do not* put ointment on a burn unless a healthcare provider tells you to do so.
- *Do not* put any medicine or household product on a burn unless a healthcare provider tells you to do so.
- *Do not* put anything on the burn except a dry dressing. Do not apply butter or oil to a burn.
- *Do not* break any blisters that form after the burn.

Question	Your Notes
1. *True or false* To help stop bleeding that you can see, put firm pressure on a dressing or bandage (eg, gauze) over the bleeding area. Circle your answer: True False	
2. *True or false* To care for a victim with a nosebleed, have her lean forward and place constant pressure on both sides of the nostrils for a few minutes until the bleeding stops. Circle your answer: True False	
3. *True or false* If a knife has been pushed into the victim's body, you should remove it as quickly as possible. Circle your answer: True False	
4. *True or false* If a victim falls from a height and then becomes sleepy or confused or vomits or complains of a headache, the victim may have a head injury. Circle your answer: True False	
5. *True or false* When giving first aid for a victim with a possible broken bone or sprain, put a plastic bag filled with ice on the injured area with a towel between the ice bag and the skin for up to 20 minutes. Circle your answer: True False	
6. *True or false* To give first aid for a small burn on the arm, cool the burn with cold but not ice cold water. Circle your answer: True False	

During the course you will have practice sessions and you will be asked to refer to the following.

Bleeding You Can See

During the practice session, participants work in pairs and take turns role-playing the victim and rescuer.

Victim	Rescuer
Bleeding from the arm	"I'm trained in first aid. May I help you?"
Agrees that the rescuer can treat him or her	• Gives victim gauze dressing and asks victim to apply pressure over bleeding area while rescuer puts on gloves. • Applies pressure over gauze. • Adds more gauze and applies pressure. • Applies bandage over dressing to maintain pressure.

Shock

During the practice session, participants work in pairs and take turns role-playing victim and rescuer. The victim is lying down and is asked by the rescuer to describe his or her signs of shock according to the following script.

Victim	Rescuer
"I'm cold, weak, and dizzy."	"My name is _____ and I'm trained in first aid. May I help you? How do you feel?"
"Yes, please help me." The victim then checks that the rescuer performs correct actions. Do not interrupt the rescuer. Wait until the rescuer has finished and then point out if the rescuer has missed a step or done something incorrectly.	• Asks someone to phone the company emergency response number (or 911). • Raises the victim's feet about the level of the heart unless there is pain or a leg injury. • Covers the victim with a blanket. • Tells the victim that help is on the way.

Environmental Emergencies

Bites and Stings

Case Example

You and your co-workers are working in a public park. One co-worker suddenly stops, bends down to look at something, and calls out, "Look at this! There's a big raccoon under this bush!" He then screams, and you realize that the raccoon has bitten his hand.

Would you know what to do?

What You Will Learn

By the end of this section you should be able to list the first aid actions for bites and stings.

Animal and Human Bites

Although many bites are minor, some may break the skin. Both animal and human mouths have many germs. When a bite breaks the skin, the wound can bleed and may become infected from the germs in the human's or animal's mouth. Bites that do not break the skin usually are not serious.

Actions for Animal and Human Bites

Follow these steps when giving first aid to a victim with an animal or a human bite:

Step	Action
1	Make sure the scene is safe for you and the victim.
2	Stay away from any animal that is acting strangely. An animal with rabies can bite again. (See "Important: Rabies" on the next page.)
3	For animal bites, phone or send someone to phone your emergency response number (or 911) and get the first aid kit.
4	Put on personal protective equipment.
5	Clean the victim's wound with running water (and soap if available).
6	Stop any bleeding with pressure.

(continued)

Step	Action
7	Report all animal bites to the police or an animal control officer. Describe • The animal • How the bite happened • The location of the animal when last seen
8	For all bites that break the skin, call the victim's healthcare provider because the victim might need shots or other medicine to treat the bite.
9	If there is a bruise or swelling, place an ice bag wrapped in a towel on the bite for up to 20 minutes.

> ### Important: Stopping Severe Bleeding
>
> If there is severe bleeding that will not stop, apply pressure and treat the injury like a major cut or scrape.

> ### Important: Rabies
>
> Assume that an animal has rabies if
>
> - The animal attacks without being provoked
> - The animal behaves in an unusual manner (for example, if a usually friendly dog attacks)
> - The animal is a skunk, raccoon, fox, bat, or other wild animal
> - You are not sure

Case Example (continued)

At the beginning of this section, you read the following Case Example:

You and your co-workers are working in a public park. One co-worker suddenly stops, bends down to look at something, and calls out, "Look at this! There's a big raccoon under this bush!" He then screams, and you realize that the raccoon has bitten his hand.

You read the following question: Would you know what to do?

Now you know what to do.

When you run over, you see that the raccoon is slowly backing off. You think that the raccoon may be rabid because it is acting strangely. You ask a third co-worker to phone your company's emergency response number (or 911) and get the first aid kit. You ask if you can help, and when he agrees, you help your co-worker clean the wound by washing his hand with running water from a hose. There is slight bleeding, which you stop with pressure. Trained help arrives and takes your co-worker to the hospital. You immediately call the police and report that a raccoon that may have rabies is in the park.

Snakebites

Case Example

While you are working at a construction site, you are called to help a co-worker who has been bitten on the leg by a snake. The snake has disappeared.

Would you know what to do?

Type of Snake

If a snake bites someone, it is helpful to be able to identify the snake. Sometimes you can identify the snake from its bite mark or behavior. *If you aren't sure whether a snake is poisonous, assume that it is.*

The following lists the signs of poisonous snakebites:

- Progressive pain at the bite area
- Swelling of the bite area
- Nausea, vomiting, sweating, and weakness

Actions for Snakebites

Follow these steps for a snakebite:

Step	Action
1	Be careful around a wounded snake: • Back away and go around the snake. • If a snake has been killed or hurt by accident, do not handle it. A snake might bite even when severely hurt or close to death. • If the snake needs to be moved, use a long-handled shovel. • If you don't need to move it, it is best to leave it alone.
2	Phone or send someone to phone your emergency response number (or 911) and get the first aid kit.
3	Ask another adult to move any other people inside or away from the area.
4	Put on personal protective equipment.
5	Ask the victim to be still and calm.
6	Tell the victim not to move the part of the body that was bitten.
7	Gently wash the bite area with running water (and soap if available).
8	If a coral snake bit the victim, apply mild pressure by wrapping a bandage comfortably tight. You should still be able to slip or fit a finger under the bandage around the entire length of the arm or leg. *Note: Do not* wrap the bite area with a dressing if any other snake caused the bite.

For information on coral snakes, refer to the CD.

Do Not

When you give first aid for snakebite

- *Do not* apply cold or ice.
- *Do not* apply suction.
- *Do not* cut the wound.
- *Do not* wrap the wound tightly.
- *Do not* use local electric shock.

Case Example (continued)

At the beginning of this section, you read the following Case Example:

While you are working at a construction site, you are called to help a co-worker who has been bitten on the leg by a snake. The snake has disappeared.

You also read this question: Would you know what to do?

Now you know what to do.

You ask someone to phone your company's emergency response number (or 911) and get the first aid kit. You make sure that the snake is not nearby and that the scene is safe for you and the victim. You ask if you may help, and the victim agrees. Then you ask the victim to lie very still and not to move his leg. You put on protective gloves when the first aid kit arrives. You wash the bite area gently with running water from a hose. You do not know whether the snake was poisonous, so you do not put a pressure dressing on the bite. You wait with the victim until trained help arrives and takes over.

Insect, Bee, and Spider Bites and Stings

Case Example

The gardener at your workplace suddenly cries out that a bee has stung her. She asks you to help. She complains that her face feels hot and "tight" and that she has tightness across the chest. She is also having trouble breathing. You notice that her face is red and beginning to look puffy. You hear a whistling noise when she breathes.

Would you know what to do?

Insect, Bee, and Spider Bites and Stings

Usually insect and spider bites and stings cause only mild pain, itching, and swelling at the bite.

Some insect bites can be serious and even fatal if

- The victim has a bad allergic reaction to the bite or sting
- Poison (venom) is injected into the victim (for example, from a black widow spider or brown recluse spider)

Actions for Insect, Bee, and Spider Bites and Stings

Follow these steps when giving first aid to a victim with an insect or spider bite or sting:

Step	Action
1	Make sure the scene is safe for you and the victim.
2	Phone or send someone to phone your company's emergency response number (or 911) and get the first aid kit if • The victim has signs of a bad allergic reaction (see "Actions for a Bad Allergic Reaction" on page 29). • The victim tells you that he or she has a bad allergic reaction to insect bites or stings
3	If a bee stung the victim • Look for the stinger. Bees are the only insects that may leave their stingers behind. • Scrape away the stinger and venom sac using something with a dull edge such as a credit card.
4	Wash the bite or sting area with running water (and soap if possible).
5	Put an ice bag wrapped in a towel or cloth over the bite or sting area to help reduce swelling.
6	Watch the victim for at least 30 minutes for signs of a bad allergic reaction (see below).

Do Not

Do not pull the stinger out with tweezers or your fingers.
Squeezing the venom sac can release more poison (venom).

Signs of a Bad Allergic Reaction

Some people can have a bad allergic reaction to insect bites, especially bee stings. People who have had bad allergic reactions to insect bites often have an epinephrine pen and know how to use it. They often wear medical identification jewelry.

Signs of a bad allergic reaction are

- Trouble breathing
- Swelling of the tongue and face
- Fainting

Actions for a Bad Allergic Reaction

Follow these steps for a bad allergic reaction:

Step	Action
1	Phone or ask someone to phone your company's emergency response number (or 911) and get the first aid kit.
2	Help the victim get the epinephrine pen and use it if your state and workplace allow you to do so (See "How to Use an Epinephrine Pen" on page 31).
3	If the victim stops responding, start the steps of CPR if you know how. (See the section "CPR and AED.")

Case Example (continued)

At the beginning of this section, you read the following Case Example:

The gardener at your workplace suddenly cries out that a bee has stung her. She complains that her face feels hot and "tight" and says that she has tightness across the chest. She is also having trouble breathing. You notice that her face is red and beginning to look puffy. You hear a whistling noise when she breathes.

You also read the following question: Would you know what to do?

Now you know what to do.

You ask the gardener if she has ever had an allergic reaction. She tells you that she is allergic to bee stings and that she has an epinephrine pen prescribed by her doctor in her car. You tell one co-worker to get the victim's epinephrine pen from the victim's car. You tell another co-worker to phone your company's emergency response number (or 911) and get the first aid kit.

When the co-worker returns with the epinephrine pen from the victim's car, you help the gardener to give herself an epinephrine injection. After several minutes the swelling, chest tightness, and wheezing lessen. You take out the stinger and venom sac by scraping the edge of a credit card along the skin. You then wash the area with soap and water and put an ice bag wrapped in a towel over the sting area. You tell the gardener that she is going to be fine.

Signs of Poisonous Spider and Scorpion Bites and Stings

The following lists the signs of poisonous spider and scorpion bites and stings. Some of the signs may vary depending on the type of bite or sting:

- Severe pain at the site of the bite or sting
- Muscle cramps
- Headache
- Fever
- Vomiting
- Breathing problems
- Seizures
- The victim does not respond

Actions for Spider and Scorpion Bites and Stings

Follow these steps for a spider or scorpion bite or sting:

Actions for Nonpoisonous Spider and Other Bites and Stings	Actions for Poisonous Spider and Scorpion Bites and Stings
1. Wash the bite with running water (and soap if available). 2. Put an ice bag wrapped in a towel or cloth on the bite or sting.	1. Make sure the scene is safe for you and the victim. 2. Phone your emergency response number (or 911) or the poison control center immediately and get the first aid kit. 3. Wash the bite with running water (and soap if available). 4. Put an ice bag wrapped in a towel or cloth on the bite. 5. If the victim stops responding, start the steps of CPR if you know how (see "CPR and AED").

Ticks

Ticks are found on animals and in wooded areas. They attach themselves to exposed body parts. Many ticks are harmless. Some carry serious diseases, like Lyme disease.

If you find a tick (Figure 31), remove it as soon as possible. The longer the tick stays attached to a person, the greater the person's chance of catching a disease.

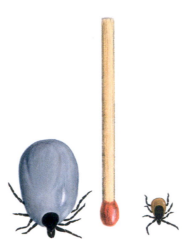

Figure 31. Ticks. Left tick is engorged; match is to show the size of ticks.

Actions for Tick Bites

Follow these steps for a tick bite:

Step	Action
1	Grab the tick by its mouth or head as close to the skin as possible with tweezers or a tick-removing device. Try to avoid pinching the tick.
2	Lift the tick straight out without twisting or squeezing its body. If you lift the tick until the victim's skin tents and wait for several seconds, the tick may let go.
3	Wash the bite with running water (and soap if available).
4	See a healthcare provider if you are in an area where Lyme disease occurs. If possible, place the tick in a plastic bag and give it to the healthcare provider.

Do Not

The following are the *wrong* actions to take when trying to remove a tick:

- *Do not* use petroleum jelly.
- *Do not* touch the tick with your bare hands.
- *Do not* use fingernail polish.
- *Do not* use rubbing alcohol.
- *Do not* use a hot match.
- *Do not* use gasoline.
- *Do not* twist or jerk the tick.

 For a map of areas affected by Lyme disease, refer to the CD.

What You Will Learn

By the end of this section you should be able to

- List the signs of a heat-related emergency
- List the first aid actions for a heat-related emergency
- List the signs of a cold-related emergency
- List the first aid actions for a cold-related emergency

Heat-Related Emergencies

Victims exposed to heat can experience heat-related emergencies. To avoid heat-related emergencies:

- Dress appropriately for the weather
- Make sure to drink plenty of fluids during hot weather

Case Example

On a very hot and humid day a worker for a landscaping company complains that she feels as if she has the flu. You notice that she is sweating. She complains that she is thirsty, tired, and sick to her stomach and has a headache.

Would you know what to do?

Signs and Actions for Heat-Related Emergencies

Heat-related emergencies can range from mild to life-threatening. You must recognize and give first aid for heat-related emergencies early because a victim with mild signs can get worse quickly and develop potentially life-threatening problems, such as heatstroke.

Many of the signs of a heat-related emergency are similar to those of the flu.

The following table shows signs and actions for heat-related emergencies and heatstroke:

Signs	Actions
Heat-Related Emergency • Muscle cramps • Sweating • Headache • Nausea • Weakness • Dizziness	1. Move the victim to a cool or shady area. 2. Loosen or remove tight clothing from the victim. 3. Encourage the victim to drink water if the victim can sit up and swallow. 4. Sponge or spray the victim with cool (*not ice cold*) water and fan the victim. 5. Phone or ask someone to phone your emergency response number (or 911) immediately if there are any signs of heatstroke. Continue to cool the victim until the victim's behavior is normal again or until trained help arrives and takes over. 6. If the victim stops responding or does not get better, phone your emergency response number (or 911) and start the steps of CPR if you know how (see the section on CPR).
Heatstroke • Confusion or strange behavior • Vomiting • Inability to drink • Red, hot, and dry skin (the victim may stop sweating) • Shallow breathing, seizures, or no response	1. Phone or ask someone to phone your emergency response number (or 911). 2. Move the victim to a cool or shady area. 3. Loosen or remove tight clothing. 4. Sponge or spray the victim with cool (*not ice cold*) water and fan the victim. Continue to cool the victim until the victim's behavior is normal again or until trained help arrives and takes over. 5. If the victim stops responding, start the steps of CPR if you know how (see the section on CPR).

Do Not

Do not ignore signs of a heat-related emergency. Symptoms of heat-related emergencies often get worse if left untreated. Mild heat-related signs are a warning that the victim may get worse unless you take action!

Do Not

- *Do not* wait to begin cooling the victim until trained help arrives and takes over. Every minute counts!
- *Do not* continue cooling the victim once the victim's behavior is normal again. Unnecessary cooling could lead to low body temperature (hypothermia).
- *Do not* put rubbing alcohol or anything other than water onto the victim's skin.
- *Do not* give the victim anything to drink or eat if the victim cannot swallow or is vomiting, confused, has had a seizure, or is not responding.

Case Example (continued)

At the beginning of this discussion, you read the following Case Example:

On a very hot and humid day a worker for a landscaping company complains that she feels as if she has the flu. You notice that she is sweating. She complains that she is thirsty, tired, and sick to her stomach and has a headache.

You read this question: Would you know what to do?

Now you know what to do.

The worker wants to finish the job, but you insist that she stop and rest in a shady area. She agrees that you can help her. You sponge her face, neck, arms, and legs with cool water while you fan her. Within 20 minutes she feels much better.

Cold-Related Emergencies

Cold-related emergencies may involve only part of the body or the whole body. A cold injury to part of the body is called frostbite. Cold injury to the whole body is called low body temperature, or hypothermia.

Case Example

You work for a snow removal company. Near the end of your shift your co-worker complains that several fingers of his right hand feel cold and numb. You ask if you can help and when he agrees, you look at his hand. The tips of his right third and fourth fingers feel cold and hard.

Would you know what to do?

Frostbite

Frostbite affects parts of the body that are exposed to the cold, such as the fingers, toes, nose, and ears. Frostbite typically occurs outside in cold weather. But it can also occur inside when workers without gloves handle cold materials, such as gases under pressure.

Signs of Frostbite

- The skin over the frostbitten area is white, waxy, or grayish-yellow.
- The frostbitten area is cold and numb.
- The frostbitten area is hard, and the skin doesn't move when you push it.

Actions for Frostbite

Follow these steps for frostbite:

Step	Action
1	Move the victim to a warm place.
2	Phone or ask someone to phone your company's emergency response number (or 911) and get the first aid kit.
3	Remove tight clothing, rings, or bracelets from the frostbitten part.
4	Remove any wet clothing.
5	Do not try to thaw the frozen part if you are close to a medical facility or if you think there may be a chance of refreezing.

Case Example (continued)

At the beginning of this discussion, you read the following Case Example:

You work for a snow removal company. Near the end of your shift your co-worker complains that several fingers of his right hand feel cold and numb. You ask if you can help and when he agrees, you look at his hand. The tips of his right third and fourth fingers feel cold and hard.

You also read and thought about this question: Would you know what to do?

Now you know what to do.

You move the victim to a warm (not hot) place. You phone your company's emergency response number (or 911) and get the first aid kit. You cover the victim with the Mylar blanket to prevent heat loss, but you do not try to thaw the frostbite. The victim is transported to the local hospital. After treatment the victim's frostbite injuries heal.

Do Not

- *Do not* rub or massage the frostbite.
- *Do not* use a heating pad, stove, or fire to rewarm a frostbite.
- *Do not* thaw the frozen part if there is any chance of refreezing or if you are close to a medical facility.

Low Body Temperature (Hypothermia)

Hypothermia occurs when body temperature falls. Hypothermia is a serious condition that can cause death. A victim can develop hypothermia even when the temperature is above freezing.

Case Example

You are a park ranger. You find a hiker who has been lost in the forest for several hours. It has been snowing and he is wet. He is not wearing cold weather gear. When you find him, he's sitting on the ground and shivering. When you ask if he's OK, he seems confused and does not respond to your question.

Would you know what to do?

Signs of Low Body Temperature

Signs of low body temperature include the following:

- The victim's skin is cool to the touch.
- Shivering (only when the victim's body temperature falls a small amount but not when the body temperature is very low).
- The victim may become confused, have a change in personality, or be very sleepy or may be unconcerned about his or her condition.
- Muscles become stiff and rigid and the skin gets ice cold and blue.

As the victim's body temperature continues to drop

- The victim stops responding
- The victim's breathing slows
- It may be hard to tell whether the victim is breathing
- The victim may appear to be dead

Actions for Low Body Temperature

Follow these steps for low body temperature:

Step	Action
1	Get the victim out of the cold.
2	Remove wet clothing and pat the victim dry. Help put dry clothes on the victim if available and cover with a blanket.
3	Phone or ask someone to phone your emergency response number (or 911) and get the first aid kit and AED if available.
4	Put blankets or towels under and around the victim, and cover the victim's head but not the face.
5	If the victim stops responding, start the steps of CPR if you know how (see the section on CPR).

Case Example (continued)

At the beginning of this section, you read the following Case Example:

You are a park ranger. You find a hiker who has been lost in the forest for several hours. It has been snowing and he is wet. He is not wearing cold weather gear. When you find him, he's sitting on the ground and shivering. When you ask if he's OK, he seems confused and does not respond to your question.

Would you know what to do?

You read and thought about this question: "Would you know what to do?"

Now you know what to do.

You quickly transport the hiker to your first aid room. You bring him inside and lay him on his back. You gently remove his cold, wet clothing, wrap him in a dry blanket, and cover him, including his head, with additional blankets and the Mylar blanket from the first aid kit. You phone your emergency response number (or 911) and stay with the victim until trained help arrives and takes over.

> **FYI: Shivering**
>
> - Shivering protects the body by producing heat.
> - Shivering stops when the body becomes very cold.

> **FYI: Rewarming the Victim**
>
> If you are far from medical care, you can start to rewarm a victim. Place the victim near a heat source and place containers of warm, but not hot, water in contact with the skin. It is important to get the victim to medical care as soon as possible.

Poison Emergencies

Poisons

According to the American Association of Poison Control Centers, a poison is anything someone swallows, breathes, or gets in the eyes or on the skin that causes sickness or death if it gets into or on the body. Many products can poison people. This section will not deal with specific poisons. Instead it will cover general principles of first aid for a poisoning victim. Follow your workplace guidelines about poisonous products in your workplace.

Case Example

You work in an electronics assembly plant. You see a co-worker coughing and rubbing her eyes. She tells you that she has just splashed a cleaning liquid on her face and asks if you will help her.

Would you know what to do?

What You Will Learn

By the end of this section you should be able to tell the steps for giving first aid for poisoning.

Scene Safety for Poison Emergencies

If you think someone may have been exposed to a poison, you must make sure the scene is safe before giving first aid. This takes a few more steps than in other first aid situations:

- Make sure the scene is safe before you approach the victim. If the scene seems unsafe, do not approach the victim. Tell everyone to move away from the victim.
  - Look for signs that warn you that poisons are nearby (Figure 32).
  - Look for spilled or leaking bottles or boxes.
  - Do not enter the scene if you see more than one poisoning victim.
- Before you approach the victim, put on appropriate protective equipment (mask, gloves, goggles, and other protective clothing).
- Try to move the victim from the scene of the poisoning if you can do so safely.
- Help the victim to go outdoors or move to an area with fresh air if possible.

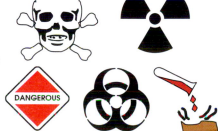

Figure 32. Look for warning signs of poisons nearby

Actions for Poison Emergencies

Follow these steps when giving first aid to someone who may have been exposed to a poison:

Step	Action
1	Make sure the scene is safe before you approach the victim. Look out for spilled or leaking bottles or boxes. • If there is a chemical spill or the victim is in an unsafe area, try to move the victim to an area with fresh air if you can do so safely. • Ask everyone to move away from the area
2	If the victim does not respond, send someone to phone your emergency response number (or 911). You stay with the victim and start the steps of CPR if you know how. Whenever possible, you should always try to use a mask when giving breaths. This is especially important if the poison is on the victim's lips or mouth.
3	If the victim responds, phone the poison control center. Tell the poison control center the name of the poison if possible.
4	Remove the poison from the victim's skin and clothing if you can do so safely. • Help the victim take off contaminated clothing and jewelry if the victim agrees. • Help the victim to a safety shower or eye wash station if the victim responds and can move. • Brush off any dry powder or solid substances from the victim's skin with your gloved hand (Figure 33). • Run water over the skin, eyes, and other contaminated areas of the victim's body for at least 20 minutes or until trained help arrives and takes over. Ask the victim to blink as much as possible while rinsing his or her eyes.
5	If you can identify the poison, send someone to get the Material Safety Data Sheet (MSDS) (see "FYI: Material Safety Data Sheets").
6	When you know the name of the poison, call the poison control center for instructions on giving first aid for poisoning. You should keep the telephone number of the poison control center in your first aid kit. To contact the poison control center: • Check the front cover of the phone book for the telephone number (800-222-1222), or go to the following website: *www.aapcc.org*. • In many communities the 911 dispatcher can connect you with the poison control center.

FYI: Material Safety Data Sheets

Worksites should have an MSDS (Material Safety Data Sheet) for each poison at the worksite. You should know where the MSDS is at your worksite.

The MSDS provides a description of how a specific poison can be harmful. This information can be very helpful at the worksite. It can also be useful to the poison control center for identifying a poison and its effects.

Unfortunately the MSDS usually provides little information about first aid actions. According to the American Association of Poison Control Centers, some of the first aid actions listed in the MSDS or on the label of the poison may be outdated.

You will probably receive additional training on the MSDS during the "Right to Know" training your workplace provides.

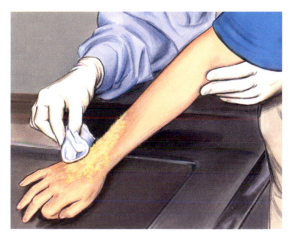

Figure 33. Brush off any dry powder or solid substances from the victim's skin with your gloved hand.

Important: Washing the Affected Area

Remember that it is very important to wash the poison off the victim using lots of water as soon as possible.

Important: Poison in an Eye

If only one eye is affected, make sure the eye with the poison in it is the lower eye as you rinse the eyes (Figure 34). Make sure you do not rinse the poison into the unaffected eye.

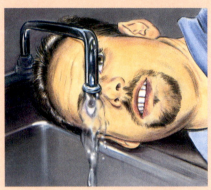

Figure 34. Help the victim wash his eyes under running water or at an eye wash station.

Case Example (continued)

At the beginning of this section, you read the following Case Example:

You work in an electronics assembly plant. You see a co-worker coughing and rubbing her eyes. She tells you that she has just splashed a cleaning liquid on her face and asks if you will help her.

You read this question: Would you know what to do?

Now you know what to do.

You help the co-worker to a safety shower. She washes the chemical from her face. You send another co-worker to phone your company's emergency response number (or 911) and get the first aid kit. The plant safety officer comes to help and has the MSDS for the cleaning liquid. The plant safety officer calls the poison control center for advice on first aid actions. When trained help arrives and takes over, she gives them the MSDS and information from the poison control center.

Do Not

- *Do not* give the victim anything by mouth unless you have been told to do so by trained help or the poison control center. This includes water, milk, syrup of ipecac, and activated charcoal.
- *Do not* rely on only the first aid instructions on the label of the bottle, can, or box.
- *Do not* apply any ointments or lotions to the skin.

FYI: Calling the Poison Control Center

When you call the poison control center, try to have the following information ready:

- What is the name of the poison? Can you describe it if you cannot name it?
- How much poison did the victim touch, breathe, or swallow?
- About how old is the victim? What is the victim's approximate weight?
- When did the poisoning happen?
- How is the victim feeling or acting now?

The following table lists general groups of poisons and other possibly dangerous substances. These poisons can enter the body by swallowing, breathing, or touching. This information is for reference only. It does not include all possible classifications or examples of all poisonous substances. The first aid rescuer is not expected to memorize these.

Classification	Examples of Poisons
Plants	Dieffenbachia Foxglove Poison ivy Poison sumac Poison oak Philodendron
Gases	Carbon monoxide Propane Methane and natural gas
Corrosives/acids	Pool cleaner Metal-cleaning solution Chlorine Ammonia
Hydrocarbons	Enamel paint Diesel fuel or gasoline Lighter fluid Turpentine
Household products	Drain cleaners Oven cleaners Toilet bowl cleaners Disinfectants Laundry detergents Bleach Pesticides and insecticides Alcoholic beverages Rubbing alcohol Furniture polish Gasoline, kerosene Antifreeze Windshield cleaner
Personal care products	Mouthwash Perfume and cologne Nail polish and polish remover
Medicines/vitamins	Nonprescription medicines, including aspirin, acetaminophen, ibuprofen, antacids, laxatives, vitamins Prescription medicines
Other chemicals	Glues and adhesives Soldering flux

Test Questions: Environmental Emergencies

Question	Your Notes
1. *True or false* You should watch a victim for at least 30 minutes after the victim has been bitten by an insect, a bee, or a spider because the victim may develop signs of a bad allergic reaction. Circle your answer: True False	
2. *True or false* A victim with low body temperature will have cool skin and may shiver or become confused. Circle your answer: True False	
3. *True or false* A victim with heatstroke will have red, hot, and dry skin and may be confused or have strange behavior. Circle your answer: True False	
4. *True or false* When a victim is having a heat-related emergency, you should move the victim to a cool place and sponge or spray the victim with cool water and fan the victim. Circle your answer: True False	

CPR and AED

Adult CPR

What You Will Learn

By the end of this section you should be able to give CPR to an adult.

Ages for Adult CPR

Adult CPR is for victims 8 years of age and older.

Overview

If you know *when* to phone your emergency response number (or 911) and *how* to give compressions and breaths, your actions may save a life. In this course you will learn the basic steps of CPR first. Then you will put these steps together in order.

There are basic steps in giving CPR:

- Doing compressions
- Giving breaths that make the chest rise

Compressions

One of the most important parts of adult CPR is compressions. When you give compressions, you pump blood to the brain and heart. You will learn more about where compressions fit in the sequence of CPR later.

Actions for Compressions

Follow these steps to give compressions to adults:

Step	Action
1	Kneel at the victim's side.
2	Make sure the victim is lying on his back on a firm, flat surface. If the victim is lying facedown, carefully roll him onto his back.
3	Quickly move or remove clothes from the front of the chest that will get in the way of doing compressions and using an AED.
4	Put the heel of one hand on the center of the victim's chest between the nipples (Figure 35A). Put the heel of your other hand on top of the first hand (Figure 35B).
5	Push straight down on the chest 1½ to 2 inches with each compression. Push hard and fast.
6	Push at a rate of 100 compressions a minute.
7	After each compression, release pressure on the chest to let it come back to its normal position.

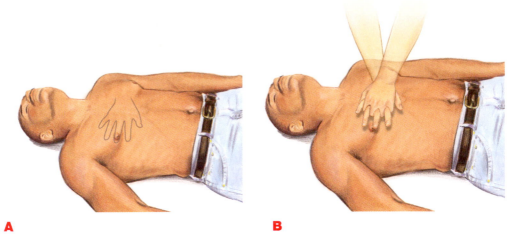

A   **B**

Figure 35. Chest compressions. **A**, Put the heel of one hand on the center of the chest between the nipples. **B**, Put the other hand on top of the first hand.

> ### *Important*
>
> These things are important to remember when doing CPR:
>
> - Push hard and push fast.
> - Push at a rate of 100 times a minute.
> - After each compression, release pressure on the chest to let it come back to its normal position.

Open the Airway

When giving CPR you must give the victim breaths that make the chest rise. Before giving breaths, you must open the airway with the head tilt–chin lift.

Performing the Head Tilt–Chin Lift

Follow these steps to perform a head tilt–chin lift (Figure 36):

Step	Action
1	Tilt the head by pushing back on the forehead.
2	Lift the chin by putting your fingers on the bony part of the chin. Do not press the soft tissues of the neck or under the chin.
3	Lift the chin to move the jaw forward.

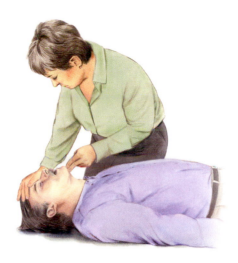

Figure 36. Open the airway with a head tilt–chin lift.

Giving Breaths

Your breaths give oxygen to someone who cannot breathe on his own.

Actions for Giving Breaths

Follow these steps to give breaths:

Step	Action
1	Hold the airway open with a head tilt–chin lift (Figure 36).
2	Pinch the nose closed.
3	Take a normal breath and cover the victim's mouth with your mouth, creating an airtight seal (Figure 37).
4	Give 2 breaths (blow for 1 second each). Watch for chest rise as you give each breath.

Figure 37. Give 2 breaths.

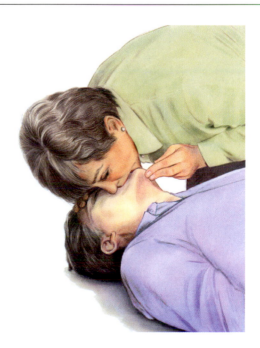

Compressions and Breaths

When you give CPR, you do sets of 30 compressions and 2 breaths. Try not to interrupt chest compressions for more than a few seconds. For example, don't take too long to give breaths or use the AED.

Putting It All Together

You have learned compressions and breaths for an adult. To put it all together in the right order, follow these steps.

Make Sure the Scene Is Safe

Before you give CPR, make sure the scene is safe for you and the victim (Figure 38). For example, make sure there is no traffic in the area that could injure you. You do not want to become a victim yourself.

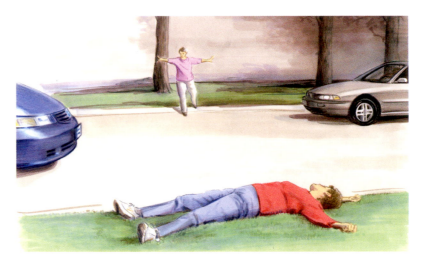

Figure 38. Make sure the scene is safe.

Check for Response

Check to see if the victim responds before giving CPR. Kneel at the victim's side. Tap the victim and shout, "Are you OK?" (Figure 39).

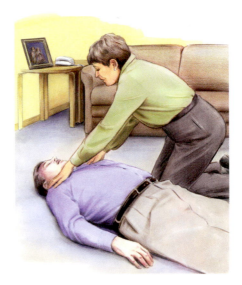

Figure 39. Check for response.

Get Help

If the victim does not respond, it is important to get help on the way as soon as possible. Follow these steps to call for help:

Step	Action
1	If the victim does not respond, yell for help. If someone comes, send that person to phone your emergency response number (or 911) and get the AED if available.
2	If no one comes, leave the victim to phone your emergency response number (or 911) and get the AED if available (Figure 40). Return to the victim and start the steps of CPR.

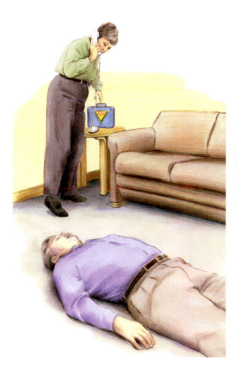

Figure 40. Phone your emergency response number (or 911) and get the AED if available.

Check Breathing

Once you have checked the victim for a response, you must check to see if the victim is breathing normally.

Step	Action
1	Open the victim's airway with a head tilt–chin lift.
2	Check to see if the victim is breathing normally (take at least 5 seconds but no more than 10 seconds) (Figure 41). • Put your ear next to the victim's mouth and nose. • **Look** to see if the chest rises. • **Listen** for breaths. • **Feel** for breaths on your cheek.

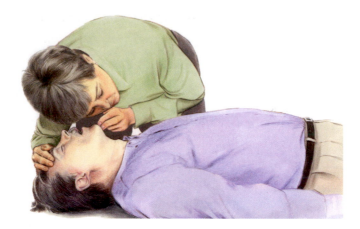

Figure 41. Look, listen, and feel for normal breathing.

Special Situations

Gasps Are Not Breaths

In the first few minutes after sudden cardiac arrest, a victim may only gasp.

Gasping is *not* breathing.

> **Important**
>
> If the victim gasps when you open the airway to check breathing, continue the steps of CPR. The victim is likely to need all the steps of CPR.

If the First Breath Does Not Go In

If you give a victim a breath and it does not go in, you will need to re-open the airway with a head tilt–chin lift before giving the second breath. After you give 2 breaths, you will give 30 compressions. You will repeat the sets of 30 compressions and 2 breaths until the AED arrives, the victim starts to move, or trained help takes over. Trained help could be someone whose job is taking care of people who are ill or injured such as an EMS responder, nurse, or doctor.

Side Position

If the victim is breathing normally but is not responding, roll the victim to his side and wait for trained help to take over (Figure 42). If the victim stops moving again, you will need to start the steps of CPR from the beginning.

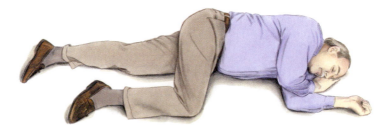

Figure 42. Side position.

The following table summarizes the steps for adult CPR:

Step	Action
1	Make sure the scene is safe.
2	Make sure the victim is lying on his back on a firm, flat surface. If the victim is lying facedown, carefully roll him onto his back.
3	Kneel at the victim's side. Tap and shout to see if the victim responds.
4	If the victim does not respond, yell for help. • If someone comes, send that person to phone your emergency response number (or 911) and get the AED if available. • If no one comes, leave the victim to phone your emergency response number (or 911) and get the AED if available. After you answer all the dispatcher's questions, return to the victim and start the steps of CPR.
5	Open the airway with a head tilt–chin lift.
6	Check to see if the victim is breathing normally (take at least 5 seconds but no more than 10 seconds). • Put your ear next to the victim's mouth and nose. • **Look** to see if the chest rises. • **Listen** for breaths. • **Feel** for breaths on your cheek.
7	If there is no normal breathing, give 2 breaths (1 second each). Watch for chest rise as you give each breath.
8	Quickly move or remove clothes from the front of the chest that will get in the way of doing compressions and using an AED.
9	Give 30 compressions at a rate of 100 a minute and then give 2 breaths. After each compression, release pressure on the chest to let it come back to its normal position.
10	Keep giving sets of 30 compressions and 2 breaths until the AED arrives, the victim starts to move, or trained help takes over.

Review Questions

1. The correct rate for giving compressions is _____ compressions a minute.
2. For adult CPR you give sets of _____ compressions and _____ breaths.
3. When giving CPR how long should each breath take?
   a. 1 second
   b. 3 seconds
   c. 4 seconds

What You Will Learn

By the end of this section you should be able to give CPR to a child.

Ages for Child CPR

For purposes of this course, a child is 1 to 8 years of age.

Overview

While some steps for giving CPR to an adult and child are similar, there are a few differences:

- When to phone your emergency response number (or 911)
- Amount of air for breaths
- Depth of compressions
- Number of hands for compressions

When to Phone Your Emergency Response Number (or 911)

If you are alone, do 5 sets of 30 compressions and 2 breaths **before** leaving the victim to phone your emergency response number (or 911). This is different from adult CPR, where you phone first.

Amount of Air for Breaths

Breaths are very important for children who do not respond. When giving breaths to children, be sure to open the airway and give breaths that make the chest rise, just as for adults. For small children you will not need to use the same amount of air for breaths as for larger children or adults. However, each breath should still make the chest rise.

Depth of Compressions

When you push on a child's chest, press straight down ⅓ to ½ the depth of the chest (Figure 43).

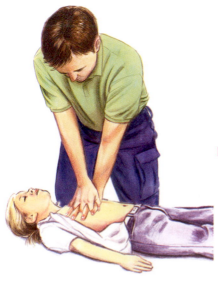

Figure 43. Two-handed chest compressions.

Number of Hands for Compressions

You may need to use only 1 hand for compressions for very small children (Figure 44). Whether you use 1 hand or 2 hands, it is important to be sure to push straight down ⅓ to ½ the depth of the chest.

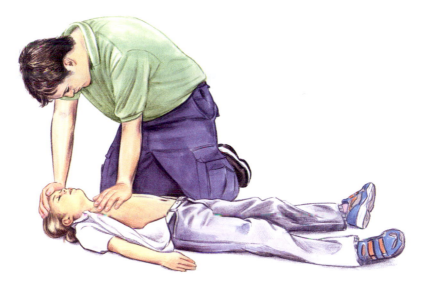

Figure 44. One-handed chest compressions.

Summary of Steps for Child CPR

The following table shows the steps for giving CPR to a child 1 to 8 years of age.

Step	Action
1	Make sure the scene is safe.
2	Make sure the victim is lying on her back on a firm, flat surface. If the victim is lying facedown, carefully roll her onto her back.
3	Kneel at the victim's side. Tap and shout to see if the victim responds.
4	If the victim does not respond, yell for help. • If someone comes, send that person to phone your emergency response number (or 911) and get the AED if available. • If no one comes, stay with the child and start the steps of CPR.
5	Open the airway with a head tilt–chin lift.
6	Check to see if the victim is breathing (take at least 5 seconds but no more than 10 seconds). • Put your ear next to the victim's mouth and nose. • **Look** to see if the chest rises. • **Listen** for breaths. • **Feel** for breaths on your cheek.
7	If the child is not breathing, give 2 breaths (1 second each). Watch for chest rise as you give each breath.
8	Quickly move or remove clothes from the front of the chest that will get in the way of doing compressions and using an AED.

(continued)

Step	Action
9	Give 30 compressions at a rate of 100 a minute and then give 2 breaths. After each compression, release pressure on the chest to let it come back to its normal position.
10	After 5 sets of 30 compressions and 2 breaths, if someone has not done this, phone your emergency response number (or 911) and get an AED if available.
11	After you answer all of the dispatcher's questions, return to the child and start the steps of CPR.
12	Keep giving sets of 30 compressions and 2 breaths until an AED arrives, the victim starts to move, or trained help takes over.

Special Situations

When giving CPR to children 1 to 8 years of age, you handle special situations, such as re-opening the airway if the first breath does not go in and the side position, the same way as you do for adults.

Review Questions

1. When giving compressions to a child, press down _____ to _____ the depth of the chest.

2. True or false: If you are alone with a child who does not respond, you should give 5 sets of 30 compressions and 2 breaths before phoning your emergency response number (or 911).

Use of Mask—Adult/Child

Using a Mask

During CPR there is very little chance that you will catch a disease. Some regulatory agencies, including the Occupational Safety and Health Administration (OSHA), require that certain rescuers use a mask when giving breaths in the workplace (Figure 45). You may also want to use a mask or other barrier device when giving CPR to victims outside the workplace who are not family members.

Masks are made of firm plastic and fit over the victim's mouth or mouth and nose. You may need to put the mask together before you use it.

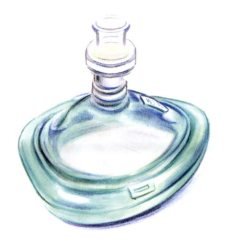

Figure 45. Mask for giving breaths.

Actions for Giving Breaths With a Mask

Follow these steps to give breaths using a mask:

Step	Action
1	Kneel at the victim's side.
2	Put the mask over the victim's mouth and nose.
3	Tilt the head and lift the chin while pressing the mask against the victim's face. It is important to make an airtight seal between the victim's face and the mask while you lift the chin to keep the airway open.
4	Give 2 breaths. Watch for chest rise as you give each breath (Figure 46).

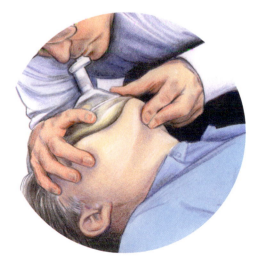

Figure 46. Giving breaths with a mask.

FYI: Masks With Pointed Ends

If the mask has a pointed end

- Put the narrow end of the mask at the top (bridge) of the nose.
- The wide end should cover the mouth.

Using AEDs

What You Will Learn

By the end of this section you should be able to

- Tell what an AED does
- Tell when you might use an AED
- List the steps for using an AED
- Tell how to give CPR and use an AED

Overview

AEDs are accurate and easy to use. After very little training, most people can operate an AED. Giving CPR right away and using an AED within a few minutes will increase the chances of saving the life of someone with sudden cardiac arrest.

What an AED Does

An automated external defibrillator (AED) is a machine with a computer inside (Figure 47). An AED can

- Recognize cardiac arrest that requires a shock
- Tell the rescuer when a shock is needed
- Give a shock if needed

An AED may give an electric shock to the heart. This can stop the abnormal heart rhythm and allow a normal heart rhythm to return.

The AED will use visual and audible prompts to tell the rescuer the steps to take. There are many different brands of AEDs, but the same simple steps operate all of them.

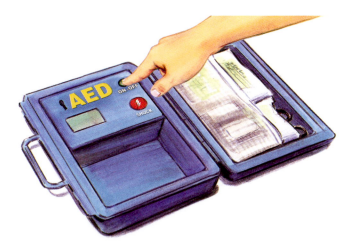

Figure 47. An automated external defibrillator (AED).

FYI: AEDs and Infants

There is currently not enough data for the AHA to recommend for or against using AEDs in infants less than approximately 1 year of age.

When You Might Use an AED

A victim who does not respond may have an abnormal heart rhythm that stops the heart from pumping blood. You will use an AED on a victim 1 year of age and older only when that victim does not respond and is not breathing.

- For victims 8 years of age and older, start CPR right away and use an AED as soon as it is available.

- For victims 1 to 8 years of age, perform 5 sets of 30 compressions and 2 breaths or about 2 minutes of CPR before attaching and using the AED.

FYI: AED Pads

Some AEDs can deliver a smaller shock dose for children if you use child pads or a child key or switch. If the AED can deliver this smaller shock dose, use it for children 1 to 8 years of age. If the AED cannot give a child dose, you can use the adult pads and give an adult shock dose for children 1 to 8 years of age.

For victims 8 years of age and older, always use the larger adult pads and adult dose—DO NOT use child pads or a child dose for a victim 8 years of age and older. You should know how to operate the AED in your workplace and know if it can provide a child dose and how to deliver that dose for a child.

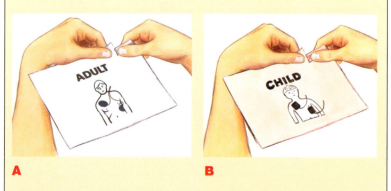

A **B**

Figure 48. AED pads. **A,** Adult pads. **B,** Child pads.

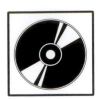

For more information on choosing the AED pads or system, refer to the CD.

Steps for Using an AED

Use the same simple steps to operate all AEDs:

Step	Action
1	**Turn the AED on.** Push the button or open the lid (Figure 49). Follow the visual and audible prompts.
2	**Attach pads** (Figure 50).
3	**Allow the AED to check the heart rhythm.** Make sure no one touches the victim (Figure 51).
4	**Push the SHOCK button if the AED tells you to do so** (Figure 52). Make sure no one touches the victim. If a shock is delivered, start the steps of CPR right after shock delivery.

Use the AED fast. For adult victims the time from arrival of the AED to first shock should be less than 90 seconds.

If the AED does not tell you to give a shock, follow the AED visual and audible prompts. Be ready to resume CPR if needed.

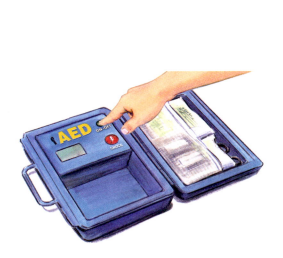

Figure 49. Turn on the AED.

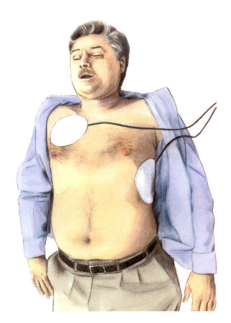

Figure 50. Attach pads.

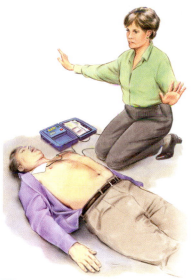

Figure 51. Clearing the victim.

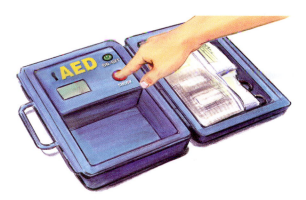

Figure 52. Press SHOCK button if needed.

Attaching Pads

Follow these steps when attaching pads:

Step	Action
1	Choose the correct pad (adult vs child) for size/age of victim (Figure 48).
2	Open the AED pad package and peel away the plastic backing.
3	Attach the sticky side of the pads directly to the victim's bare chest (Figure 50). The picture on the pad will show you where to put the pads.

Clearing the Victim

You must "clear" the victim before the AED analyzes the victim's heart rhythm or gives a shock dose to the victim. To clear the victim, look around to make sure no one touches the victim when the AED prompts you to clear (Figure 51).

Special Situations

Special situations will change the way you use an AED.

Water

Do not deliver a shock when a victim is

- Lying in water
- Covered with water (for example, the victim is covered with sweat or has just been pulled from a swimming pool)

Water may cause the shock to flow over the skin from one pad to the other. If that happens, energy won't go to the heart.

If you give a shock in water, the AED also might shock the rescuer.

Step	Action
1	Move the victim away from standing water.
2	Quickly wipe the victim's chest before you attach the pads.

FYI: AEDs and Small Amounts of Water

If the victim is lying in a small puddle of water or snow but the chest is not covered with water, you can give shocks.

Medicine Patch

You should not put an AED pad over a medicine patch. The patch may block some of the shock dose so that some of the energy does not reach the heart. Also, giving a shock over the patch may burn the victim.

Step	Action
1	If a child or adult has a medicine patch in the same place where you would attach the AED pad, take the medicine patch off while wearing gloves.
2	Quickly wipe the chest where the patch was before you put on the pad.

Implanted Pacemaker or Defibrillator

Some children or adults may have an implanted pacemaker or defibrillator. These devices make a hard lump under the skin of the chest or in the abdomen. The lump is smaller than a deck of cards. You should not put an AED pad over this lump because the implanted device may block delivery of the shock to the heart.

Step	Action
1	Look for a lump under the skin of the chest that looks smaller than a deck of cards.
2	If you see this lump where the pads should go, put the pads at least 1 inch away from the lump.

Hairy Chest

If a victim has a hairy chest, the AED pads may stick to the hair instead of the skin on the chest. If this happens, the AED will not be able to check the victim's heart rhythm or deliver a shock. The AED will prompt you to check the pads.

Step	Action
1	If the pads stick to the hair instead of the skin, press down firmly on each pad.
2	If the AED still tells you to check the pads, quickly pull off the pads to remove the hair.
3	If a lot of hair still remains where you will put the pads, shave the area with the razor in the AED carrying case.
4	Put on a new set of pads. Follow the AED visual and audible prompts.

FYI: AEDs in the Community

The American Heart Association supports placing AEDs throughout the community in lay rescuer AED programs. AEDs are placed in many public places where large numbers of people gather, such as sports stadiums, airports, airplanes, and an increasing number of worksites.

AED programs usually are directed by a healthcare provider and are linked with the local EMS system. AED rescuers, such as police, security guards, trained first aid providers, and volunteers should be trained in CPR and the use of an AED.

You can increase the chance of survival for a victim of sudden cardiac arrest if you give the victim CPR right away and use an AED within a few minutes.

For more information on taking care of an AED, refer to the CD.

You can get this information at your workplace after the course.

Key Points From My Workplace Emergency Response Policies and Procedures

How to access the workplace emergency response system:

Phone:_____

Where the AED (if available) is located: _____

What changes do you need to make to use the AED on a child?

____Use "child" pads

____Insert a "child" key or turn a "child" switch

____Other: _____

Masks used at the workplace (check one):

____Yes ____ No

Other key points:

_____

_____

_____

Review Questions

1. True or false: You can use adult AED pads on a child if child pads are not available.

2. Which of the following best describes "clearing the victim"?
   a. Taking the pads off the victim's chest
   b. Making sure no one is touching the victim
   c. Moving the victim to a clear room

Infant CPR

What You Will Learn

By the end of this section you should be able to give CPR to an infant.

Ages for Infant CPR

Infant CPR is for victims from birth to 1 year of age.

Overview

While some steps for giving CPR to an infant are similar to giving CPR to an adult or child, there are a few differences:

- How to give compressions
- How to open the airway
- How to give breaths
- How to use a mask
- How to check for response

You will first learn the skills of CPR for the infant that are different from adult and child CPR. Then you will learn to put all the steps together in the correct order.

Compressions

As with CPR for the adult and child, compressions are a very important part of infant CPR. Compressions pump blood to the brain and heart.

Actions for Compressions

Follow these steps to give compressions to an infant:

Step	Action
1	Place the infant on a firm, flat surface. If possible, place the infant on a surface above the ground, such as a table. This makes it easier to give CPR to the infant.
2	Quickly move or open clothes from the front of the chest that will get in the way of doing compressions.
3	Put 2 fingers of one hand just below the nipple line. Do not put your fingers over the very bottom of the breastbone (Figure 53).
4	Press the infant's breastbone straight down ⅓ to ½ *the depth* of the chest. Push hard and fast.
5	Repeat at a rate of 100 compressions a minute.
6	After each compression, release pressure on the chest to let it come back to its normal position.

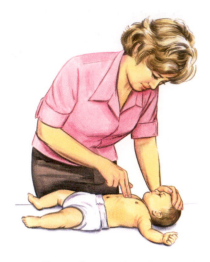

Figure 53. Put 2 fingers just below the nipple line.

> **Important**
>
> These things are important to remember when doing CPR:
>
> - Push hard and push fast.
> - Push at a rate of 100 times a minute.
> - After each compression, release pressure on the chest to let it come back to its normal position.

Open the Airway

When giving CPR you must give the infant breaths that make the chest rise. Before giving breaths you must open the airway with the head tilt–chin lift.

Performing the Head Tilt–Chin Lift

When you open an infant's airway, use the head tilt–chin lift (Figure 54). When tilting an infant's head, do not push it back too far because it may block the infant's airway.

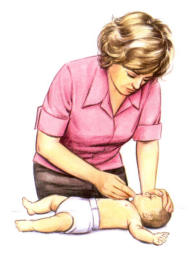

Figure 54. Use the head tilt-chin lift.

Giving Breaths

Breaths are very important for infants who are not breathing or do not respond. Your breaths give an infant oxygen when the infant cannot breathe on his own. You will not have to give as large a breath to an infant as you give to a child or an adult.

Actions for Giving Breaths

Follow these steps to give breaths to infants:

Step	Action
1	Hold the infant's airway open with a head tilt–chin lift.
2	Take a normal breath and cover the infant's mouth and nose with your mouth, creating an airtight seal (Figure 55).
3	Give 2 breaths (blow for 1 second each). Watch for chest rise as you give each breath.

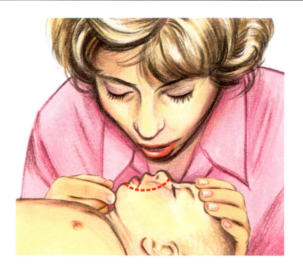

Figure 55. Cover the infant's mouth and nose with your mouth.

FYI: Tips for Giving Breaths

If your mouth is too small to cover the infant's mouth and nose, put your mouth over the infant's nose and give breaths through the infant's nose. (You may need to hold the infant's mouth closed to prevent air from escaping through the mouth.)

Check for Response Check to see if the infant responds before giving CPR. Tap the infant's foot and shout, "Are you OK?" (Figure 56).

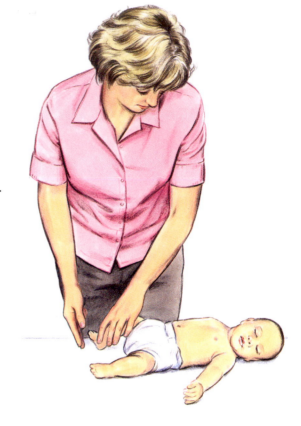

Figure 56. Check for response.

Get Help If the infant does not respond, it is important to get help on the way as soon as possible. Follow these steps to get help:

Step	Action
1	If the infant does not respond, yell for help. If someone comes, send that person to phone your emergency response number (or 911).
2	If no one comes, stay with the infant and continue the steps of CPR.

Special Situation If you give an infant a breath and it does not go in, you will need to re-open the airway with a head tilt–chin lift before giving the second breath.

Summary of Steps for Infant CPR

The following table summarizes the steps for infant CPR:

Step	Action
1	Make sure the scene is safe.
2	Tap the infant's foot and shout to see if the infant responds.
3	If the infant does not respond, yell for help. • If someone comes, send that person to phone your emergency response number (or 911). • If no one comes, stay with the infant to start the steps of CPR.
4	Place the infant on a firm, flat surface. If possible, place the infant on a surface above the ground, such as a table.
5	Open the airway with a head tilt–chin lift.
6	Check to see if the infant is breathing (take at least 5 seconds but no more than 10 seconds). • Put your ear next to the infant's mouth and nose. • **Look** to see if the chest rises. • **Listen** for breaths. • **Feel** for breaths on your cheek.
7	If the infant is not breathing, give 2 breaths (1 second each). Watch for chest rise as you give each breath.
8	Quickly move or open clothes from the front of the chest that will get in the way of doing compressions.
9	Give 30 compressions at a rate of 100 a minute and then give 2 breaths. After each compression, release pressure on the chest to let it come back to its normal position.
10	After 5 sets of 30 compressions and 2 breaths, if someone has not done this, leave the infant and phone your emergency response number (or 911).
11	After you answer all of the dispatcher's questions, return to the infant and start the steps of CPR.
12	Keep giving sets of 30 compressions and 2 breaths until the infant starts to move or trained help takes over.

FYI: Taking the Infant With You to Phone for Help

If the infant is not injured and you are alone, after 5 sets of 30 compressions and 2 breaths, you may carry the infant with you to phone your emergency response number (or 911).

1. The correct rate for giving compressions is _____ compressions a minute.
2. For infant CPR you give sets of _____ compressions and _____ breaths.
3. When giving CPR to an infant, how long should each breath take?
   a. 1 second
   b. 3 seconds
   c. 4 seconds

Use of Mask—Infant

Using a Mask

Using a mask for an infant is the same as for an adult or child except for a couple of things:

- Any mask should cover the infant's nose and mouth but should not cover the infant's eyes.

- If you do not have an infant mask, follow the recommendations of the manufacturer of the mask you are using.

Infant Choking

What You Will Learn

By the end of this section you should be able to show how to help a choking infant.

Signs of Choking

When food or an object such as a toy gets in the airway, it can block the airway. Infants can easily choke if they put small things in their mouths.

Choking can be a frightening emergency. If the block in the airway is severe, you must act quickly to remove the block. If you do, you can help the infant breathe.

The signs of choking are the same for adults, children, and infants except that the infant will not use the choking sign.

How to Help a Choking Infant

When an infant is choking and suddenly cannot breathe or make any sounds, you must act quickly to help get the object out by using back slaps and chest thrusts.

Follow these steps to relieve choking in an infant:

Step	Action
1	Hold the infant facedown on your forearm. Support the infant's head and jaw with your hand. Sit or kneel and rest your arm on your lap or thigh.
2	Give up to 5 back slaps with the heel of your free hand between the infant's shoulder blades (Figure 57).
3	If the object does not come out after 5 back slaps, turn the infant onto his back. Move or open the clothes from the front of the chest only if you can do so quickly. You can push on the chest through clothes if you need to.
4	Give up to 5 chest thrusts using 2 fingers of your free hand to push on the breastbone in the same place you push for compressions (Figure 58). • Support the head and neck. • Hold the infant with one hand and arm, resting your arm on your lap or thigh.
5	Alternate giving 5 back slaps and 5 chest thrusts until the object comes out and the infant can breathe, cough, or cry, or until the infant stops responding.

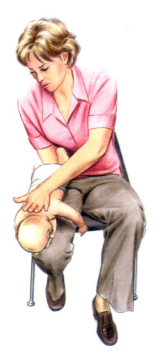

Figure 57. Give up to 5 back slaps with the heel of your hand.

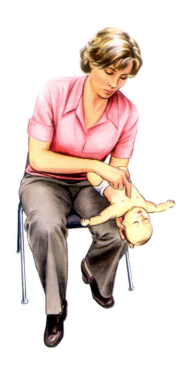

Figure 58. Give up to 5 chest thrusts.

When to Stop Back Slaps and Chest Thrusts

Stop back slaps and chest thrusts if

- The object comes out
- The infant begins to breathe, cough, or cry
- The infant stops responding

Actions for a Choking Infant Who Stops Responding

If you cannot remove the object, the infant will stop responding. When the infant stops responding, follow these steps:

Step	Action
1	Yell for help. If someone comes, send that person to phone your emergency response number (or 911). Stay with the infant to start the steps of CPR.
2	Place the infant on a firm, flat surface. If possible, place the infant on a surface above the ground, such as a table.
3	Start the steps of CPR.
4	Every time you open the airway to give breaths, open the infant's mouth wide and look for the object. If you see an object, remove it with your fingers. If you do not see an object, keep giving sets of 30 compressions and 2 breaths. Continue CPR until the infant starts to move or trained help takes over.
5	After about 5 cycles or 2 minutes, if you are alone, leave the infant to call your emergency response number (or 911).
6	Return to the infant and continue the steps of CPR.

Do Not

DO NOT use abdominal thrusts on an infant. Abdominal thrusts could injure an infant.

Review Questions

1. How can you help relieve choking in an infant who is responding and crying?

    a. Back slaps and chest thrusts

    b. Nothing

    c. Abdominal thrusts

2. True or false: You should try to relieve choking if an infant is coughing loudly.

Conclusion

Congratulations on taking time to attend this course. Contact the American Heart Association if you want more information on CPR, AEDs, or even first aid. You can visit *www.americanheart.org/cpr* or call 877-AHA-4CPR (877-242-4277) to find a class near you.

Even if you don't remember all the steps of CPR exactly, it is important for you to try. And always remember to phone your emergency response number (or 911). They can remind you what to do.

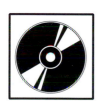

For information on signs of heart attack and stroke, as well as general anatomy and physiology, refer to the CD.

Comparison of CPR and AED Steps for Adults, Children, and Infants

CPR	Adult and Older Child (8 Years of Age and Older)	Child (1 to 8 Years Old)	Infant (Less Than 1 Year Old)
Check for response	Tap and shout		Tap the infant's foot and shout
Phone your emergency response number (or 911)	Phone your emergency response number (or 911) as soon as you find that the victim does not respond	Phone your emergency response number (or 911) after giving 5 sets of 30 compressions and 2 breaths	
Open the airway Use head tilt–chin lift	Head tilt–chin lift		Head tilt–chin lift (do not tilt head back too far)
Check breathing If the victim is not breathing, give 2 breaths that make the chest rise	Open the airway, look, listen, and feel (Take at least 5 seconds but no more than 10 seconds)		
First 2 breaths	Give 2 breaths (1 second each)		
Start CPR	Give sets of 30 compressions and 2 breaths		
• Compression location	Center of chest between nipples		Just below the nipple line
• Compression method	2 hands	1 or 2 hands	2 fingers
• Compression depth	1½ to 2 inches	⅓ to ½ depth of chest	
• Compression rate	100 a minute		
• Sets of compressions and breaths	30:2		
To relieve choking	Abdominal thrusts		Back slaps and chest thrusts (no abdominal thrusts)
AED • Turn the power on (or open the case)	Use AED as soon as it arrives	Use AED after 5 sets of 30 compressions and 2 breaths	
• Attach pads to the victim's bare chest	Use adult pads	Use child pads/key/switch or adult pads	
• Allow the AED to check the heart rhythm	Clear and analyze		
• Push the SHOCK button if prompted by the AED	Clear and shock		
• Time from arrival of AED to first shock	Less than 90 seconds		

Heartsaver First Aid Course
Adult/Child CPR and AED
Student Practice Sheet

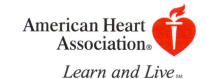

American Heart Association®

Learn and Live sm

Step	Critical Performance Steps	Details
1	_____ Check for response	Tap victim and ask if the person is "all right" or "OK," speaking loudly and clearly.
2	_____ Tell someone to phone your emergency response number (or 911) and get an AED	Tell someone to perform **both** actions.
3	_____ Open airway using head tilt–chin lift	Place palm of one hand on forehead. Place fingers of other hand under the lower jaw to lift the chin. Obvious movement of the head back toward the hand on the forehead.
4	_____ Check breathing	Place face near the victim's nose and mouth to listen and feel for victim's breath. Look at chest. Take at least 5 seconds but no more than 10 seconds.
5	_____ Give 2 breaths (1 second each)	Seal your mouth over victim's mouth and blow. Your exhaled breaths should take 1 second each. Reposition the head if chest does not rise.
6	_____ Bare victim's chest and locate CPR hand position	Move or remove clothing from front of victim's chest. Place heel of one hand in the center of chest, between the nipples.
7	_____ Deliver first cycle of 30 compressions at the correct rate	Give 30 compressions in less than 23 seconds. Push hard; push fast; let chest return to normal between compressions.
8	_____ Give 2 breaths (1 second each)	Seal your mouth over victim's mouth and blow. Your exhaled breaths should take 1 second each. Reposition the head if chest does not rise.

PRACTICE SHEETS

Adult/Child CPR and AED Student Practice Sheet (continued)

Step	Critical Performance Steps	Details
AED Arrives		
AED 1	_____ Turn AED on	Stop CPR and press button to turn AED on (or make sure that AED case is open if your AED has an automatic-on feature).
AED 2	_____ Select proper pads and place pads correctly	Recognize the difference between adult pads and child pads: • Select the proper pad size for the manikin • Apply the pads to the chest as pad diagrams and/or AED instructions show
AED 3	_____ Clear victim to analyze	Show a visible sign of clearing the victim and a spoken indication of clearing the victim: "Clear! Stay clear of victim!" or similar words with an obvious gesture to make sure all are clear.
AED 4	_____ Clear victim to shock/press shock button	Show a visible sign of clearing the victim and a spoken indication of clearing the victim: "Clear! Stay clear of victim!" or similar words with an obvious gesture to make sure all are clear. Press shock button when prompted and after clearing. For adult victim, time from arrival of AED to first shock must be less than 90 seconds.
Continue CPR		
9	_____ Resume CPR: deliver second cycle of compressions using correct hand position	Place heel of one hand in the center of chest, between the nipples. Do 30 compressions. Push hard; push fast; let chest return to normal between compressions.
10	_____ Give 2 breaths (1 second each)	Seal your mouth over victim's mouth and blow. Your exhaled breaths should take 1 second each. Reposition the head if chest does not rise.
11	_____ Deliver third cycle of compressions of adequate depth with chest returning to normal	Do 30 compressions. Push hard; push fast; let chest return to normal between compressions.

Heartsaver First Aid Course
Infant CPR
Student Practice Sheet

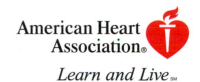

American Heart Association®

Learn and Live ℠

Step	Critical Performance Steps	Details
1	_____ Check for response	Tap infant's foot and shout loudly.
2	_____ Tell someone to phone your emergency response number (or 911)	Tell someone to phone emergency response number (or 911). (During class practice there is someone to phone 911; otherwise do 2 minutes of CPR before phoning 911.)
3	_____ Open airway using head tilt–chin lift	Push back on forehead, place fingers on the bony part of the victim's chin and lift the victim's chin. Do not press the neck or under the chin. Lift the jaw upward by bringing the chin forward. Do not push the head back too far.
4	_____ Check breathing	Place face near the victim's nose and mouth to listen and feel for victim's breath. Look at chest. Take at least 5 seconds but no more than 10 seconds.
5	_____ Give 2 breaths (1 second each) with visible chest rise	Seal your mouth over victim's nose and mouth and blow. Your exhaled breaths should take 1 second each. You should be able to see the chest rise twice.
6	_____ Bare victim's chest and locate CPR finger position	Move or open clothing from front of victim's chest. Place 2 fingers just below the nipple line.
7	_____ Deliver first cycle of 30 compressions at the correct rate	Give 30 compressions in less than 23 seconds. Push hard; push fast; let chest return to normal between compressions.
8	_____ Give 2 breaths (1 second each) with visible chest rise	Seal your mouth over victim's nose and mouth and blow. Your exhaled breaths should take 1 second each. You should be able to see the chest rise twice.
9	_____ Deliver second cycle of compressions using correct finger position	Compress chest with 2 fingers just below the nipple line. Do 30 compressions. Push hard; push fast; let chest return to normal between compressions.
10	_____ Give 2 breaths (1 second each) with visible chest rise	Seal your mouth over victim's nose and mouth and blow. Your exhaled breaths should take 1 second each. You should be able to see the chest rise twice.
11	_____ Deliver third cycle of compressions of adequate depth with chest returning to normal	Do 30 compressions. Push hard; push fast; let chest return to normal between compressions.

Heartsaver First Aid Course Evaluation

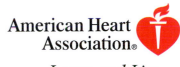

Our goal is to ensure that we are providing an effective program that meets your needs and expectations. We value your opinion and need your feedback. Please take a moment to complete this course evaluation. The administrator of this program will review your ratings and comments on the delivery, facilities, instructor, and overall satisfaction with the course.

Administration and Facilities

Date of course? _____ Who were the instructors? _____

Where was the course held? _____

Circle a number that matches your opinion on each statement.

Statement	Strongly Disagree	Disagree	Neutral	Agree	Strongly Agree
It was easy to enroll in the course.	1	2	3	4	5
I received my *Heartsaver Student Workbook* and CD in time for me to read the pre-class assignments.	1	2	3	4	5
The course facilities were adequate.	1	2	3	4	5
There was enough equipment available for everyone to practice skills with little "standing around" time.	1	2	3	4	5
The equipment was clean and in good working order.	1	2	3	4	5

Instruction

Circle a number that matches your opinion on each statement.

Statement	Strongly Disagree	Disagree	Neutral	Agree	Strongly Agree
My instructor communicated clearly.	1	2	3	4	5
My instructor answered my questions.	1	2	3	4	5

Satisfaction

Circle a number that matches your opinion on each statement.

Statement	Strongly Disagree	Disagree	Neutral	Agree	Strongly Agree
I would recommend this course to others.	1	2	3	4	5
I can apply the skills I learned.	1	2	3	4	5

Any comments you would like to make on the delivery, facilities, instructor, and overall satisfaction with the course? Please write your comments on the back of this form.

Please return your completed course evaluation to your instructor or your regional ECC office.

INDEX